Aqua Kriya yoga

M-aking
A-qua
Y-oga
A-ccessible

Camella Nair

AuthorHouse™
1663 Liberty Drive, Suite 200
Bloomington, IN 47403
www.authorhouse.com
Phone: 1-800-839-8640

©2007 Camella Nair. All rights reserved.

No part of this book may be reproduced, stored in a retrieval system, or transmitted by any means without the written permission of the author.

First published by AuthorHouse 10/18/2007

ISBN: 978-1-4343-3404-6 (sc)

Printed in the United States of America
Bloomington, Indiana

This book is printed on acid-free paper.

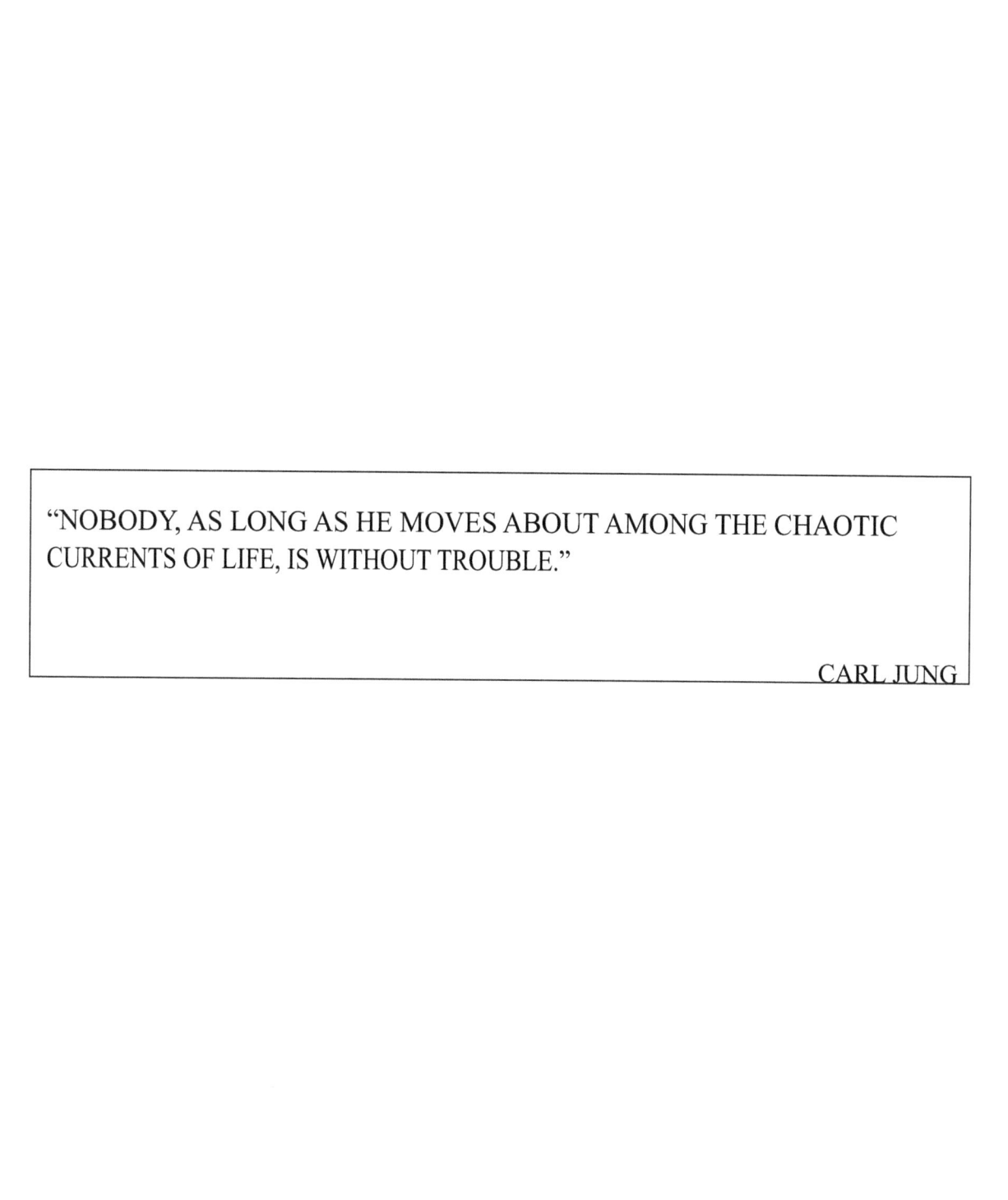

"NOBODY, AS LONG AS HE MOVES ABOUT AMONG THE CHAOTIC CURRENTS OF LIFE, IS WITHOUT TROUBLE."

CARL JUNG

Health and Safety Notice

You must take ultimate responsibility for your own well being and health. This includes being aware of your surroundings and your body's reaction to these postures. Aqua Yoga expands the opportunity for healthful exercise to many people, even those with a specific body bias. It may not be suitable, however, for a given person's unusual or advanced condition. Before you practice Aqua Yoga for the first time, please consult with a physician to make sure the activities are suitable for your situation. You should also have regular check-ups over the years, and listen to what your body tells you along the way. If you have never done yoga before it is important that you take lessons from a certified teacher and please don't overdo things. Make sure that the environment you have chosen to practice in is conducive to your health and safety and that adequate provision has been made for children requiring supervision. These postures take place in the water, so please be careful of slippery surfaces outside and inside the pool. If a movement feels uncomfortable or begins to hurt, stop and relax. In case of sharp or lasting pain, or numbness or of light-headedness, please obtain medical advice before resuming practice. Stay hydrated, but don't drink the pool water.

The benefits one gets from these yoga postures vary with each person's intensity, duration and horizon of awareness. Try not to compare your progress with others, or push yourself too hard. Enjoy each moment with a positive focused energy and I expect you too will feel the benefits of Aqua Yoga.

May you find joy in the practice.

FORWARDS

"Camella Nair's Aqua Kriya Yoga Book", is much more than a lovely book of yoga postures done in the water. This book is thoughtful, original, making Hatha Yoga safe, accessible and a source of healing for every b-o-d-y, I personally can't wait to try postures and mantra in the hot tub...very enlightening."
Lilias Folan - Internationally acclaimed yoga teacher, PBS Host and Author of "Yoga Gets Better With Age".

"Camella Nair has pioneered the use of yoga for the disabled person, using aquatics and appropriate yoga postures. From a psychological point of view, her programs have an immense impact on the self-esteem and growing confidence of her students."
William Yabroff, PhD. Professor Emeritus. Fielding Graduate Institute in Clinical Psychology.

Health and fitness books these days are nearly as abundant as autumn leaves. Every so-called expert, it seems, has written at least one or two, and the total of them is simply overwhelming. But how often in this crowded genre is there anything truly innovative and new? Most of these books are like the rest, managing merely to rewrap the same ideas, advice and techniques. Furthermore, almost none of them, no matter how stylish they may be, appears to understand or address what health and fitness are really all about: the potential to access a higher state of being.

"Camella Nair's Aqua Kriya Yoga is not only unique in the exercise field, it flows like water itself from a source of ancient wisdom that emphasizes the whole person: body, mind and soul. Here is an interweaving of powerful yogic principles, self-study, self-discipline, divine attunement - with postures that accentuate strength and flexibility, with breathing techniques that calm and center the mind, and all within a medium - water - that is fundamentally conductive to the qualities of nurture and support. One discovers more in this book than a fresh and practical approach to health improvement; one discovers a doorway to greater consciousness and transformation. Camella is steeped in the art and science of yoga, and the serious reader, student or teacher who partakes of what she offers here will realize far more in depth and personal worth than health and fitness alone."
James Conti - Manager, East West Bookstore. Mountain View. California

"I am a stroke survivor. For the last fourteen years, I have survived, and for the last fourteen years, I have been involved in therapy. I have tried and done everything. I rode a horse, had acupuncture, and massages. I stretched, worked out with weights, and I swam.

Water has been my favorite. Before my stroke (when I was active in sports), I did yoga. I loved the poses and especially the "Salute to the Sun". Now my favorite thing is practicing yoga in the water.

Why? Because I am free. The water buoyancy reduces my weight considerably;
my right side is unreliable and weak. However, in the water I can move the right
side as well as my stronger left. The water is a friendly environment for me.

Water yoga is remarkable. My instructor stresses breathing. I had forgotten what that meant. Once upon a time, when I was fully able-bodied, I knew how to breathe. Fourteen years is a long time and I forgot. Now, in the water yoga class, I am reminded and I breathe in and out, in and out. The result is a lighter, stronger me. My outer body moves freely, my internal organs enjoy the massage, and my right arm moves closer and closer to breaking out of the water. My right leg moves easier. I stretch my torso, and my whole body rejoices. I can even walk without assistance in the water. One of these days, I will transfer that ability to walking on land.

In the meantime, I look forward to my Friday class at the Saratoga YMCA with Camella showing me the way to harmony through breath and conscious movement.

I know another water teacher who reminds me that the water is my friend. With that friend's help, I can almost touch my universe."

Thomas Matola, Ph.D. Author of "Don't Pull the Plug"

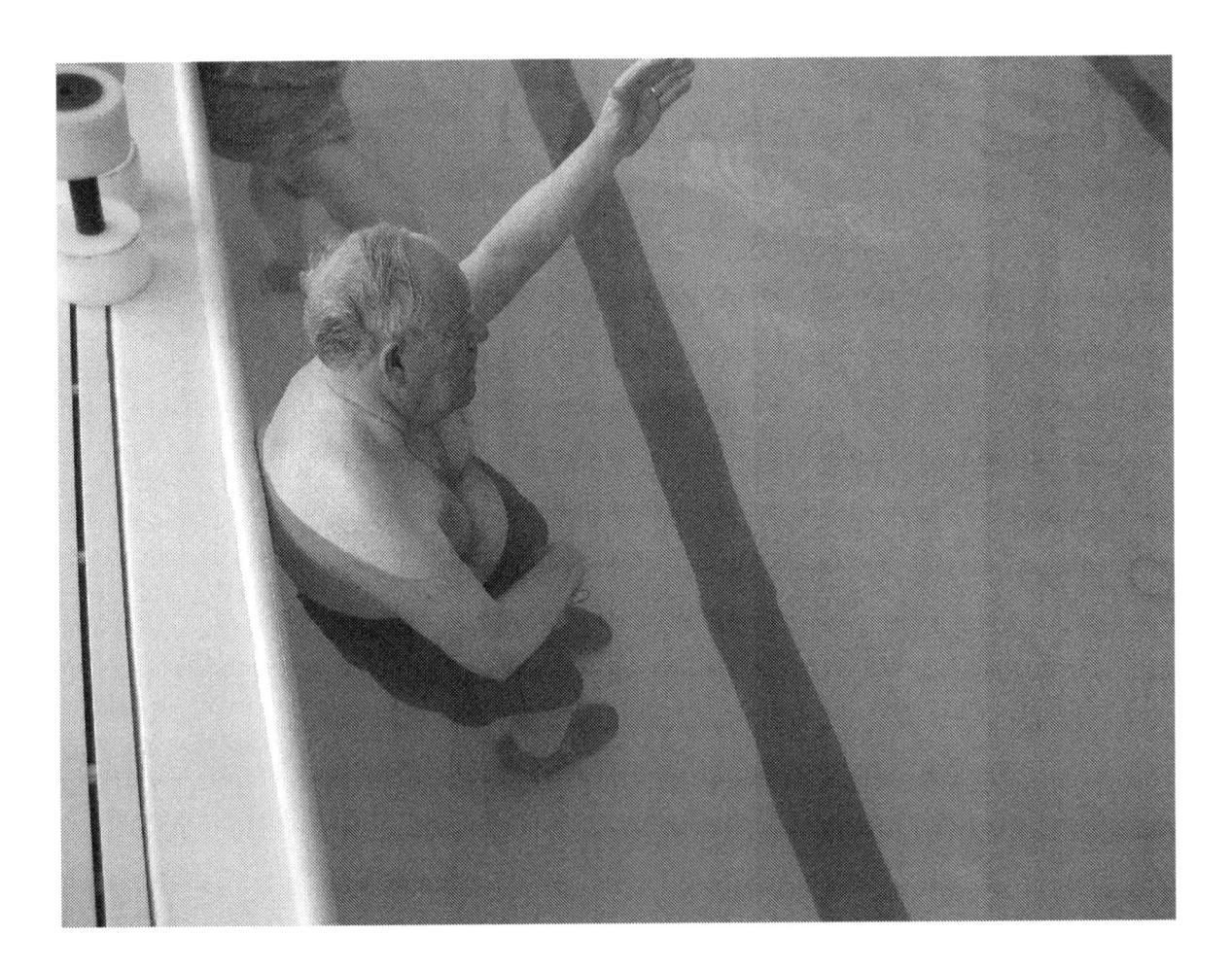

Tom working in the direction of tree pose with good arm overhead and focusing on his breathing.

Eight

"The highest good is like water.
Water gives life to the ten thousand things and
does not strive,
It flows in places men reject and so is like the Tao."
Tao Te Ching – Lao Tsu
(A New Translation by Gia Fu Feng and Jane English)

STUDENT TESTIMONIALS.

" Water yoga can change your life! As with most overweight people, I assumed that I was incapable of experiencing what yoga can do for the mind, body and spirit. With guidance from Camella, I have experienced the lengthening and strengthening of my muscles whilst learning about the importance of each breath. Not just breathing, but to breathe healing into my own body. By concentration on your breath, you can enhance your mind, and the greatest result is, you strengthen your spirit. Body size or physical fitness does not matter. If you want to live a healthy life, getting in touch with your body, mind and spirit, water yoga is for you. Relax and enjoy!"

Phyllis Belcher… Aqua Kriya Yoga Student

"For those of us who are limited on land due to injury or the healing process, Aqua Yoga is a wonderful alternative so we can stay active and not injure ourselves. I started attending the Aqua Yoga classes at the 'Y' to improve my general health and to enhance the mobility in my knees and shoulder. After six surgeries on my left knee and two on my right, typical yoga classes have been beyond me. I could not participate in the traditional yoga classes that require getting down on your knees. I also had a rotator cuff surgery a few years ago and lost some movement in my right shoulder. My doctor felt that water exercise would be a huge benefit for my general overall health.

The Aqua classes offered at the 'Y' sounded very interesting. I have had an interest in yoga for many years as a way to improve my flexibility and help me to relax. Aqua Yoga is very low impact on my joints and better yet, the warm water helps me to stretch and feel more flexible. I don't feel my knees during or after the class! With just a few weeks of classes under my belt, I can move my shoulder with more ease and with less pain than I have had in many years. The relaxation floating at the end of class is a special treat. I would recommend Aqua Yoga to anyone looking for some form of stretching and relaxation and cannot manage to participate in the gym. It is a wonderful alternative to traditional yoga."

Cindy Drew… Aqua Yoga Student

"In September 2003, I became a member of the Southwest YMCA in Saratoga, California. First, I wanted to do some lap swimming because I just love being in the water and love swimming. It's calming for me. Then, as I was looking at the schedule, I found out that there was an Aqua Yoga class every week. It got my attention. I already knew what yoga on land looked like, but Aqua Yoga was new to me. I had a feeling that it would be fun to try, but I was concerned that it might be too easy at the same time. Curiosity got me…I decided to try it that same week.

My first time was just perfect. In the water environment breathing, moving and doing yoga poses was just so relaxing. At that time, I also had sciatica problems, so being in the water permitted me to use the supporting advantage of the water environment. My leg could move without having all the weight on it, which was not the case on land. Then 1 started to think, water and yoga combined. Why not? This combination opens the door to a variety of people of all ages to explore and experience yoga's benefits. It brings about a quiet and peaceful environment, merging water with body and breath awareness. A real recipe to attain peace, balance and harmony within.

Two years later, I became a certified Yoga Instructor and started teaching Aqua Yoga. It helps me to open up the 'Yoga experience', to more people who have physical limitations and who cannot participate in a land class. Aqua Yoga has opened up my mind to teaching, and sharing yoga in, and outside the formal classroom. People just have to be willing to get their feet wet and open their minds to another level."

Julie Bleau Certified Yoga Instructor and Student

"When I was pregnant with each of my children, I enjoyed being in the water. It relieved the pressure and stress the baby put on my body. I was able to concentrate on my inner strength.

Aqua Yoga was the best way to incorporate both stress relief for my mind and body in one class. The breathing techniques performed in yoga coincided perfectly with my lamaze breathing exercises. Although I could not do all of the yoga poses due to my doctor's restrictions, I was able to stretch out my muscles that were sore from the pregnancy. After the baby was born, I still enjoy my Aqua Yoga class because it helps relieve stress, and gives me the energy to tackle motherhood."

JeAnna Weisend… Pre and Post Natal Student

NEPTUNE (God of the Sea)

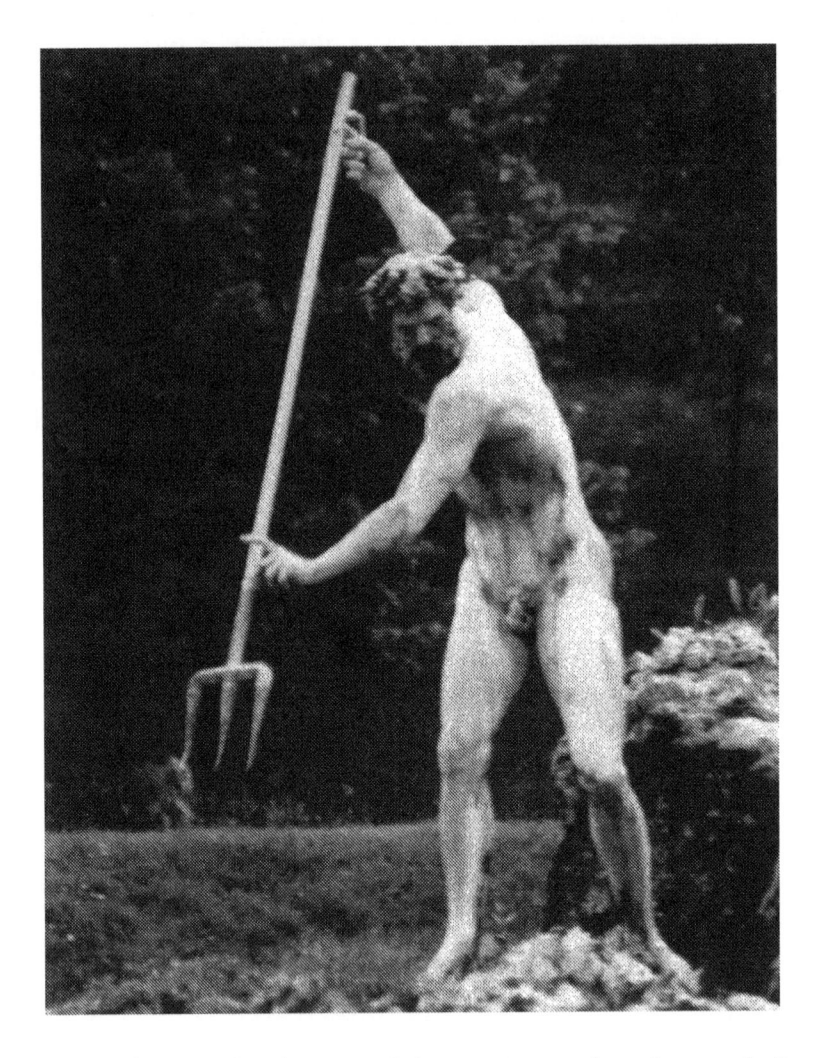

Just like Shiva (transforming force) on Land, he carries a trident that symbolizes the gunas or qualities of inertia, passionate activity, and equanimity. (tamas, rajas, sattwa)

We are made up of a mixture of all three qualities, but in yoga are trying to soften the rough edges of our personality, thus becoming more peaceful and content, (sattwa dominant)

The goal, if there be one, is to learn to live in this garden of God with Wisdom, Joy and Contentment. To become part of the solution to the problems we face in this World.

PRAJNA- ANANDA – MOKSHA
(Wisdom   Bliss   Liberation)

Neptune as a Symbol of Transformation

Shiva is the patron saint of yoga, and is the symbol of the Divine state of consciousness within us that transforms. We can improve our lives from where we are at right now. Some people want to loose weight, some to ease joint pain, some to lengthen muscles, and some to relearn how to breathe. No one's reason for coming to yoga is more valid than another. What we are trying to do in yoga, is modify and redirect the forces of nature within us, to bring about change and greater serenity and balance. We can have what we want. We just have to go about it with skillful means and self-awareness.

The way we breathe affects the way we think. As we take in and absorb more oxygen into the body, we start to feel more alive, and the knowledge of what we need to change, is revealed to us on an individual level. A problem is: the inability to seek a solution to the problem we are facing.

We live in a society where we are constantly reminded of how 'imperfect we are.' The problem is, we think we are the physical body and the thoughts in the mind. This is erroneous thinking, as we are not the physical body, nor the content of the mind. Long after the physical body dies the soul is still very much alive but just in a different form. Then we fall asleep spiritually, and forget all we have learned, until at some point, we begin the practice of searching for the meaning of life once again .We do this until we become established in it, and we connect with the Divine source. Kriya Yoga is using the energy of the mind within us to think something more positive, and less destructive to ourselves, and others. Thoughts are the seeds of action, so we should not ignore them, but learn from them.

Billions of dollars are spent on perfecting the physical body, with no real investment in trying to improve our personality. In Kriya Yoga, the physical body is only the vehicle of transformation, and as such needs to be tuned up once in a while to keep it running. If you have the body of say a Porsche, great. But a beaten up old Chevy may get you from A to B just the same. (actually, maybe faster, as it may not have such a big ego investment) Someone's real beauty comes from deep within and can be seen as an attitude to life. The greatest area for improvement is also in this area of attitude, and it is from here that the yogi learns to make better choices in life. Becoming healthier, more balanced, less judgmental and more compassionate to others. My guru says: "The greatest gift you can give to the world, is your own self-transformation."

Table of Contents

FORWARDS	vii
STUDENT TESTIMONIALS.	x
NEPTUNE (God of the Sea)	xii
Neptune as a Symbol of Transformation	xiii
The Water Element as a psychological State of Consciousness	xviii
Dedication	xix
My Background	xxi
Kriya Yoga	xxiv
About this Book	xxvii
Some benefits of practicing the Asanas in water	xxix
Typical Students	xxxi
Inclusion Yoga	xxxii
Introduction	xxxiv
Bridging the Mind and Body	1
The Lotus as a Metaphor in Yoga	3
The Churning of the Mind stuff	5
Connecting to the Inner Mermaid	8
The Breath	10
The Pool Requirements	12
The Sequencing of Asanas	13
Aqua Yoga and the Competitive Swimmer	17
The Asanas	20
Key Student Instructions	20
Poolside Teacher Notes	20
1- MOUNTAIN POSE	24
1A – Cow's Face Arms	25
2- Cat – Cow	26
3- Knee to Chest – Leg Stretch	27
4- Arms Extended Overhead	29
5- Fierce Pose	30
6-Warrior 1	31
7- Walking Warrior	33
8 – Torso lengthening pose	34
9- Stabilize shoulders	35
9A-More Shoulder Work	36
10- Warrior 2 & Half Moon	37
11- Lateral Angle Pose & Triangle Pose	39
12- Straight Leg & Reverse Twist	41
13- Horse Stance	42
14- Rainbow Shoulder Rotations	43
15- Plank Pose & Side Plank Pose	44
16 – Eagle Pose	46

17- Simple Backbend	47
18- Tree Balance	48
19- Cobra Pose	49
20- Tummy Toners	50
21- Groin Stretch & Hip Opener	51
22- Noble Seal Pose	53
23. Resting Pose or Corpse Pose	54
MORE ADVANCED WORK	55
24- Handstand	55
25 – Torpedo Scull (engaging uddiyana bandha)	57
26 – Reverse Torpedo	58
27- Poolside Arm Balance	60
28- Chakric Wheel	61
29- Monkey Stretch	62
30- Deep Twist with Shoulder Stability	63
31- Reverse Triangle Pose	64
32- Pelvic Tilt & Feet to Wall (Cat-Cow Variation)	65
33- Warrior 3 & Backbend Scull	66
34- Hip Opener & Side Bend	67
Basic Sun Salutations	69
Aqua Yoga and the Pre-Natal Student	74
Aqua Yoga whilst on Vacation	83
Aqua Yoga in the Hot Tub	91
Kriya Yoga in the Bathroom	97
Patanjali's 8 limbs of Self Transformation	100
The Water You Drink	105
Pranayama (life force control)	110
Sacred Waters	112
Aqua Yoga and Meditation	117
Acknowledgements:	123
Bibliography:	125

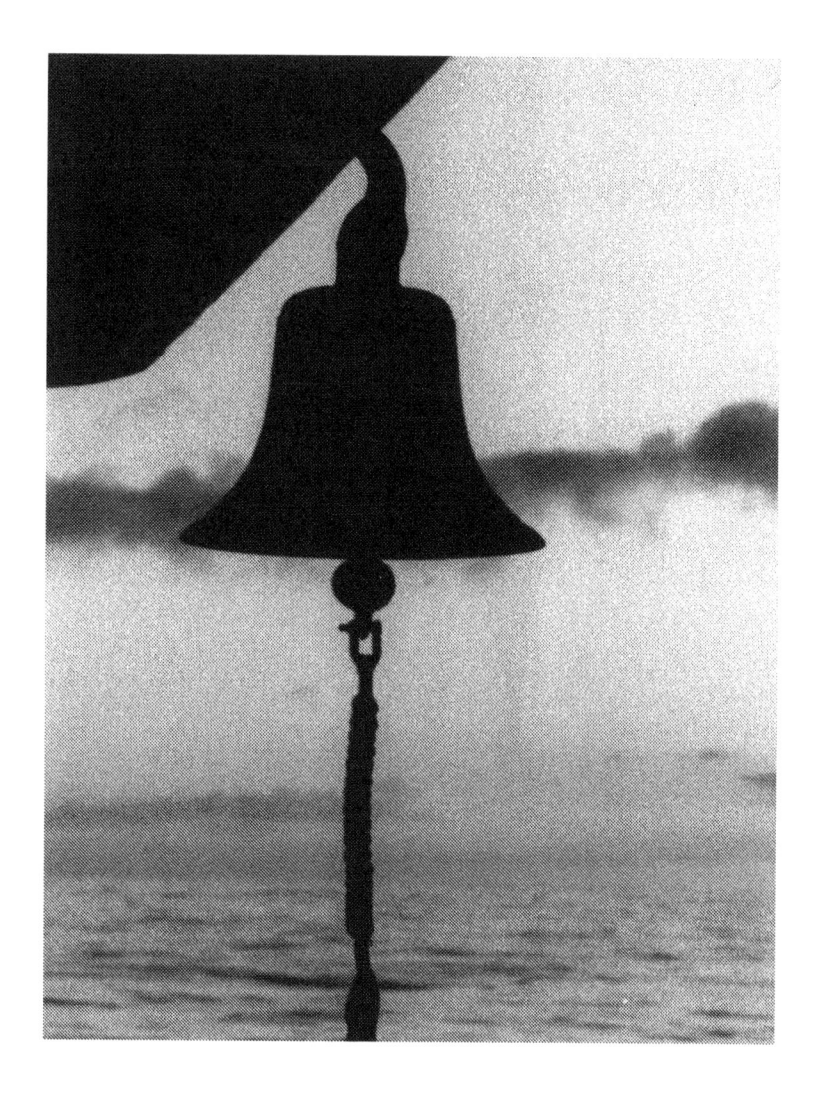

Like the power of the sea eroding and changing the landscape, with discipline and self-awareness, we can change the self- limiting thoughts that confine and very often define us.

In Shakespeare's plays, the characters emotions are traditionally symbolized by water.

" I saw him beat the surges under him
And ride upon their backs; he trod the water,
Whose enmity he flung aside, and breasted".

"The Wisdom of Shakespeare" - Peter Dawkins

The Water Element as a psychological State of Consciousness

The energy centers considered in yoga are associated with various areas within what is regarded as the subtle spine, or astral body. In our yoga practice, we are balancing these centers, which are associated with psychological urges. They either open an energy center and allow more energy in, or close an energy center, and limit the flow of energy known as Prana into it. These energy centers are known as chakras (ch as in church), and are often depicted as a flowering lotus.

The outer wheel of these chakras are where emotional energy is stored as thoughts, which are really just vibrations. The goal therefore, is to 'get' to the center of each chakra, and become more balanced.

Now, if you can close your eyes and visualize the tailbone, which probably is now close to the chair you are sitting on. This is where the root chakra, or muludhara chakra is located. It is related to the Saturn state of consciousness. Saturn when balanced is a great stabilizer, organizer, and hard worker. Those who have Capricorn as their Sun sign know this already. If this energy center or chakra, has not been balanced, then the psychological urge would be seen as a person who feels very limited, or confined and perhaps, even fearful. It is a destructive place to be emotionally, because we can feel hopeless and, or helpless. This Saturn chakra is associated with the Earth element.

We do have the tools to modify these destructive urges within us however, and we do this by balancing and lifting our energy literally to a higher state of consciousness, and into another element, which just happens to be associated with the element of water. This is located at the sacrum and is ruled by the planet Jupiter. It is associated with expansion in terms of abundance, and optimism.

On a subtle level, the energies are said to correspond to the Doctrine of Quintuplication. Each gross element is made up of just half of its pure element, say Water. The remaining half is then made up of one eighth of each of the other four elements (earth, fire, air, ether) Thus each element has an elemental dominance but is not separate from the other elements. This is a fascinating example of the matrix of consciousness we find ourselves in. Everything is connected.

In Astrology, the element of water symbolizes a force that is emotional, sensitive, and cautious. The water signs are Cancer, Scorpio and Pisces. We may have our sun, moon or ascending planet in a water sign, and the area or house that these planetary forces fall into (or life area), can be a key area in which we can find greater self-awareness, and balance. It is therefore well worthwhile studying a few basic astrological terms, such as planets, signs and houses, along with their meaning, and associated psychological urges. These can be found in most astrology books.

Imagine the Earth receiving no, or little water. It becomes parched, dry and cracks easily. Nothing can grow in it. In our yoga practice, we are focusing so much on refining our postures for a reason. To modify the subtle energies within and become more balanced. The subtle energy or Prana will flow better, and the mind will follow the Prana, thus becoming more tranquil. Very often the additional absorption of oxygen and Prana will improve memory and creativity. This, in itself makes us feel much more content about fulfilling our potential in this lifetime.

Dedication

With this book, I acknowledge the teachings, and the love passed down to me from the Kriya lineage, as revealed to me by my Guru and Paramguru,

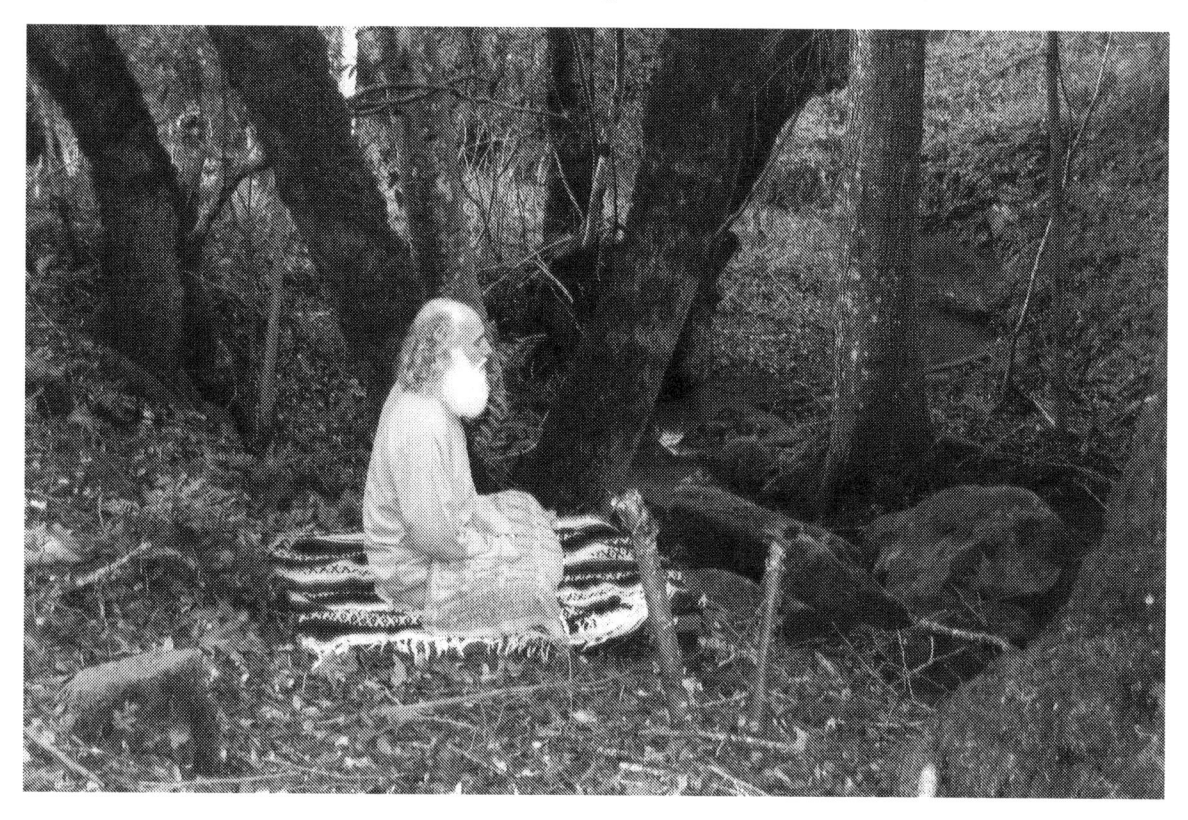

I dedicate this book to the many people out there in our society that have not yet experienced the profound sense of serenity that can be found through the practice of yoga.

Very often, people think that they have to be fit and flexible before beginning a yoga practice. This is simply not true, and I hope to dispel that myth with this book. There are many teachers who are bringing yoga to people who have a bias in the body that requires a sensitive approach or modification. Even beyond that group, there are many people that love to be in the water, but have not experienced yoga, and they too can embrace the positive changes that result from the discipline that yoga brings.

It is to this group of people that very often have a very low self-esteem about what they can achieve, that I send my deepest respect and regard. Beginners in yoga do have to work so much harder than intermediate students. Don't get discouraged. With practice, patience and perseverance, you can improve your life, and yes, you can become more fulfilled.

I am grateful to the YMCA organization for having the insight to support Aqua Yoga as part of their "physability program." This allows people who have Cerebral Palsy, Multiple Sclerosis, Parkinson' Disease, Post Stroke, Spine Injury, Arthritis, Diabetes, Post Polio, Developmental Disability, Obesity, Post Rehabilitation and many other disabling conditions to taste yoga, often for the first time.

Thanks to Eric Small for his personal account of Aqua Yoga. He was inspired by his teacher, B.K.S.Iyengar to take his yoga into the water to help overcome M.S.

Special thanks go to the model students in this book. They are a blessing in my life.

Deepest blessings go to all new students of yoga, whatever their level of ability, for the chance to move towards greater self-improvement, and even greater self-awareness.

Tat Twam Asi - That Thou Art

My Background

I have been practicing yoga for more than 25 years, after attending classes with my mother at a local community center.

What I have since discovered is that cultivating inner body length and breath control through my training in synchronized swimming, benefited my body many years prior to coming onto the yoga mat.

As humans we live in a 'bubble' that helps us to sustain our physical existence with the air that we breathe. There are many other universes beyond Earth that require different mediums to sustain their life forms. For most of us, it is challenging enough to conceive of us being a part of life in the earth's rivers, lakes and oceans.

In water, we are limited. If we put our head under water, we can only hold the breath for so long before we need to come up and take some air. Practicing breath control and self- awareness, can really help us to appreciate the gift of each breath.

I am certified as a hatha yoga instructor from the Temple of Kriya Yoga in Chicago, and also have a certification in Ayurvedic yoga from the California College of Ayurveda. I am a registered teacher with the Yoga Alliance and a member of the International Association of Yoga Therapists.

My favorite hatha teacher is Kim Schwartz, who is a teacher's teacher of exceptional ability. He taught me how to teach not only the articulation of asana, but also how to embody one's own personal practice.

I teach a variety of styles of yoga on land, including, pre-natal, vinyassa, and meditation.

I hope to be offering teacher training in Aqua Kriya Yoga in the near future.

Interested students can e-mail me at camyoga@gmail.com.

The Reflection Pond at Ickwell Bury (Bedford, England)

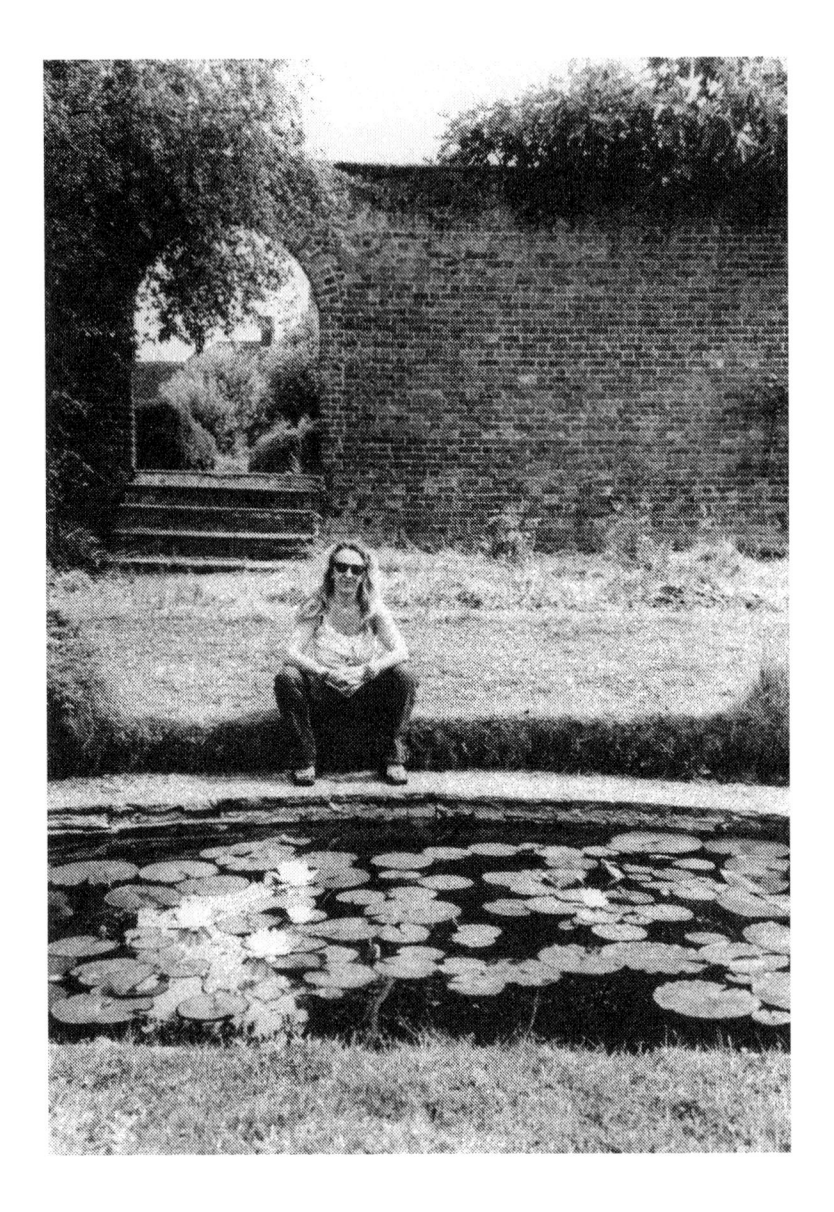

One of the most relaxing and influential yoga centers I have been to was at 'The Bury", as it was affectionately known. It used to be the Headquarters for the Yoga for Health Foundation that was pioneered by Howard Kent. They helped many people manage chronic illness such as cancer, heart problems, M.S, nervous disorders and the like.

Sadly now, the property has been taken over by land developers. A real loss for the yoga community, and therapeutic yoga in particular.

The mind when tainted cannot be purged in the
external pilgrimage places, where people bathe physically.

(Purification is of a subjective, mental disposition, and can
happen because of a seeker's action in that place, or any
other place)

The Kriya Yoga Upanishad 4:54 Translated by Goswami Kriyananda

Kriya Yoga

TAPAHA-SVADHYAYESVARA-PRANIDHANANI KRIYA-YOGAH.

Kriya Yoga it the yoga of Self-Revelation through the alchemical process of;

Self-Discipline	Tapas	(third Niyama, observance)
Self-Study	Svadhyaya	(fourth Niyama)
Attunement	Ishvara Pranidhana	(fifth Niyama)

It is the type of yoga specifically mentioned in the Yoga Sutra's, and is an incredible series of techniques and teachings that are transmitted from one generation to the next mostly in the oral tradition. From teacher to student or Guru to disciple. It is not so much about studying on an intellectual level, but coming to understand through experience, and then, embody that for yourself.

There are many organizations that have attuned to the Kriya Lineage, brought to America by Paramahansa Yogananda. No one organization is better than another. The student will merely be drawn to the organization that resonates with their soul, and their disposition. Whilst they may each have a different emphasis on the teachings, all basically share one common practice of sacred breathing techniques that rotate energy around the 12 levels of consciousness, or mansions of the soul. The physical body is the very vehicle of transformation. The transformation is a movement from unawareness to awareness, to balanced self-awareness. People often ask, "well, what type of yoga do you teach? Is it Iyengar, Ashtanga,etc?" In my heart, it is Kriya Yoga. It does have many elements to it. The precision of Iyengar for example in its physical aspect. Yet it is so much more. If you were to take a Hatha Yoga teacher, a psychologist, an astrologer, and an alchemist. Then mix them together. You would come up with a Kriya yogi. They are mystical scientists that long to discover, and understand the very meaning of life. Not what we have had downloaded into our subconscious mind by our culture and civilization, but an unbiased experience of what the earth life should be about. A Life Divine. Where we attune to all life forms, recognizing that we are all part of the same supreme source.

We come to recognize that we have been blessed with the tools to become happier and wiser, and therefore to enjoy life to the full. We just have to move, beyond our concept of who and what we think we are.

It is a way of trying to improve our lives, and thereby improving the lives of those around us, as we stop trying to put the blame of our problems "out there". To begin this process, we need to be able to look at ourselves, and our ego personality, "warts and all", and see what work needs to be done. This process begins with the breath, so we need to learn techniques that explore how, and why we breathe the way we do, and what affect it has upon our mind and the thoughts we think. The way we breathe ultimately affects the way we think. Understanding this process is a conscious Kriya, or action, and as such needs to be experienced, and not just understood intellectually.

In the physical discipline of yoga (Hatha), we can begin to understand the body more. Far easier perhaps than understanding the mechanism of the mind. The body, and whatever bias it may have, will inhibit the flow of energy, and so affect the movement of life energy or Prana in the subtle body which, in turn will affect the stability of the mind. In this case, the cycle of the breath is likely to be somewhat distorted, e.g. shorter inhale, or exhale. The body and the particular shapes we make with it, with practice, allows us greater insights as to where we are imbalanced physically, emotionally, and spiritually. It can also help us maintain and improve the body, mind complex, as we try to sustain continuity of the breath

If. And, when, the student is ready and wants to deepen their understanding further, the teacher will appear. They may be from the Kriya Lineage, or from another school of thought that helps people on the spiritual path, for there are many ways. All lead to the same goal. There is only one important one however, and that is the one that the individual has chosen as being meaningful to them. They may go to many lectures, classes and read many books, but at some point, they will choose and stick with one path, and see it to its end. It is about a lifestyle where all of the areas in our life fit together harmoniously to balance the puzzle that is life.

In the Dharma.

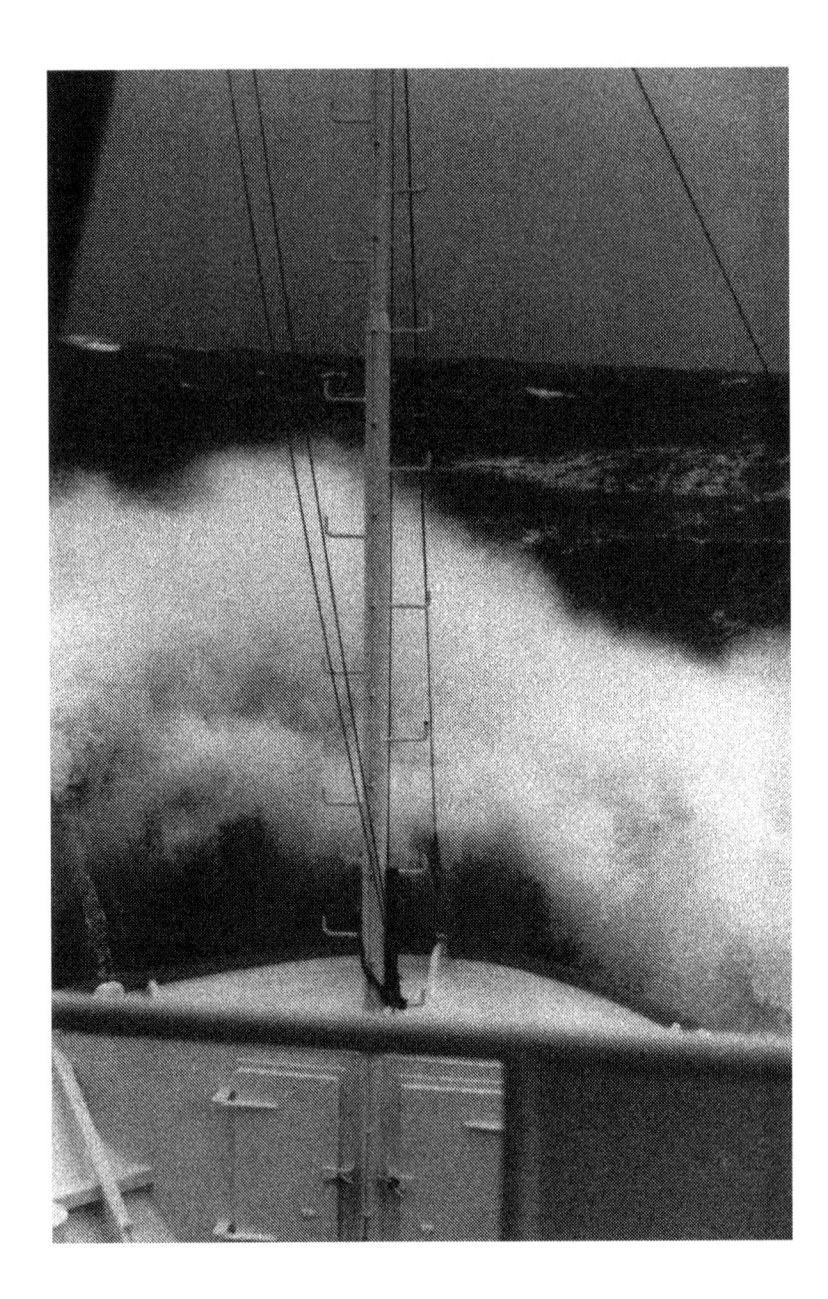

The waves crashing onto the bow of the ship are like the thoughts we bump into. We are not responsible for them, but we are responsible for what we do with them.

Our perception of water and the sea like anything else is subject to our stored memory track and our reaction to certain events. For some, the sea is claming, yet for others it is a place of misery due to past events and the fear it evokes.

About this Book

This book is for students and potential students of all levels, and the best teachers are always students. I wanted people of all levels of initiation into yoga to be able to begin practicing "Aqua Yoga", and have included lots of photographs which I hope will help to keep it simple and fun. For the 'novice', you can begin here. Gradually, if you find meaning in the practice, you will begin asking more questions about what you are trying to do, and how you can improve what you are doing. At this point, you might want to study the section on, 'Key Student Instructions', or even further refine your practice, with the 'Teacher Notes'.

For those students or yoga teachers that want to study Aqua Yoga and teach classes, this is a good reference book.

The main problem about communication, as my Guru once said, is the problem of language. How does one communicate so that people can understand what you are trying to say, and then apply that methodology or philosophy in a way that is meaningful to them?

I hope that this book will be both meaningful to students and teachers, but do recognize that there is a vocabulary in yoga that may need to be demystified for some.

The language of the kitchen for example, talks about,' beating the eggs', 'baking things blind', 'creaming together', and so forth. But how does this translate to baking a pie? What Kriya or actions need to be performed?

I have tried to keep the yoga language simple. As with everything, if you know something, it is simple, so please forgive me if I have forgotten how to think as a 'non-yogi', and did not explain something adequately. You will find basic translations on words in the many books currently available that devote a great deal of time explaining their meaning. Also, you may have an organization or teacher close by who can help you de-mystify the language. It is good to be curious and ask questions.

If you want to learn more about Kriya Yoga as a mystical science, you can visit any good book store, or go online. My personal recommendation is 'The Spiritual Science of Kriya Yoga', which you can obtain from the Temple of Kriya Yoga in Chicago, or visit www.yogakriya.org.

Yoga is about becoming more Self-aware, and if you have any doubt about any of the exercises contained within this book, you should consult your doctor or find a certified yoga instructor near-by.

It is my sincere wish that new students will experience the serenity of yoga, and improve their lives. We should find joy in our practice, and yoga is intended to be experiential, so begin from where you are, and enjoy the journey.

The best teachers are always students, but we are all teachers on some level. It could be a mother or friend at the poolside on holiday, coaching postures for fun, or a certified yoga instructor leading a scheduled class, and helping students deepen their practice. Either way, how you use the book will be subject to time, place, circumstance and the horizon of your awareness.

I hope you find greater joy through practicing.

Floating in Resting/Corpse Pose

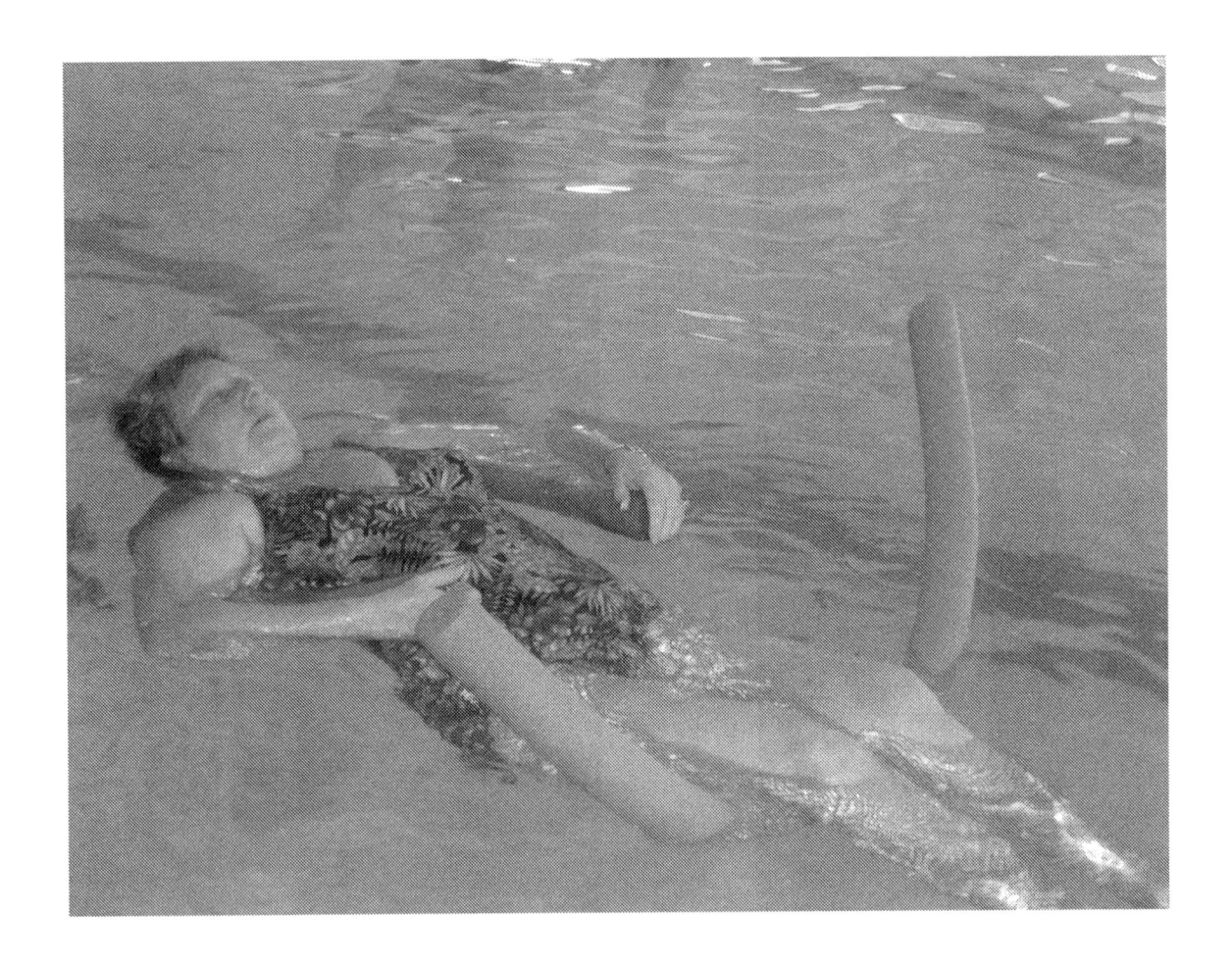

Yoga is about getting rid of our angular energy, known as emotionality.
We empty ourselves in order to fill ourselves afresh with more noble thoughts.

Some benefits of practicing the Asanas in water

The benefits of practicing the postures or asanas in water, is slightly different to those on land. The bones are not loaded in the same way for example. This can be a blessing to those suffering from arthritis or swollen joints etc. This really is thinking 'off the mat', making yoga accessible to those who would not find the practice suitable or meaningful on land. Reaching up out of the water cultivates and sustains inner body length. Generally speaking, the asanas are best articulated close to the wall, rather than in the middle of the pool. The wall offers some resistance to deepen and best of all help stabilize the asana, so that a deeper inquiry into the breath can be made.

Seniors especially seem to love being in the water. They generally feel they are less likely to hurt themselves in this environment. People after surgery and post stroke find it a nice, stimulating environment that helps them forget their bias by focusing on refining their breathing technique. This helps them cultivate a reverence for the mind, body and spirit. Take control of their lives and feel good about them-selves.

In some cases, reliving memories of summer fun as a child practicing handstands under the water, can actually help those who are having difficulty practicing these on land. It may help them gain confidence taking the hips above the shoulders. Of course one may have issues going underwater, but for some it may be meaningful.

People who are heavy, and especially "ladies in waiting", can enjoy a light sense of freedom in the water. Poses such as 'half moon', which is a wonderful body opener and balance, yet challenging on land, can be experienced in the water by many groups of students. They tend to feel they have more inner space and strength, which improves their sense of well being. The support of the water allows them to try new things without the fear of falling and hurting themselves.

I have listed many asanas that translate well to the water, but it is by no means the definitive list. Practice and experience often leads to new asanas being revealed.

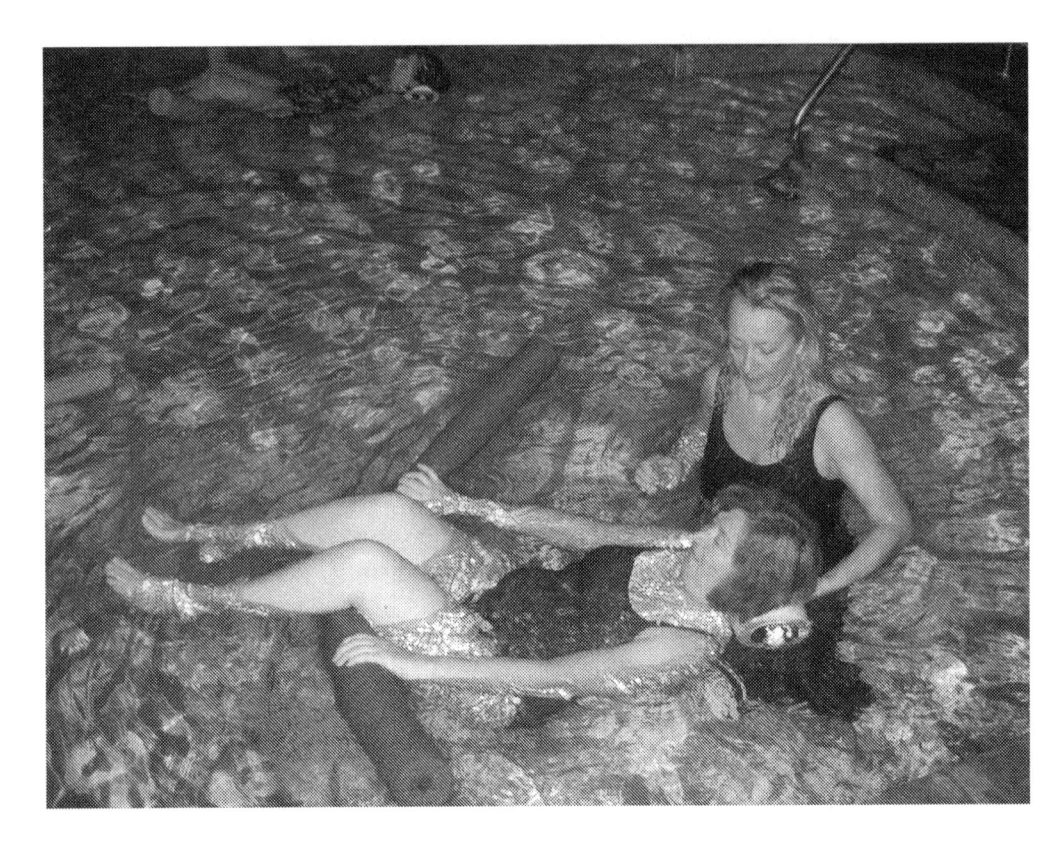

Assistance and encouragement can help the fearful student to begin to let go of resistance to change.

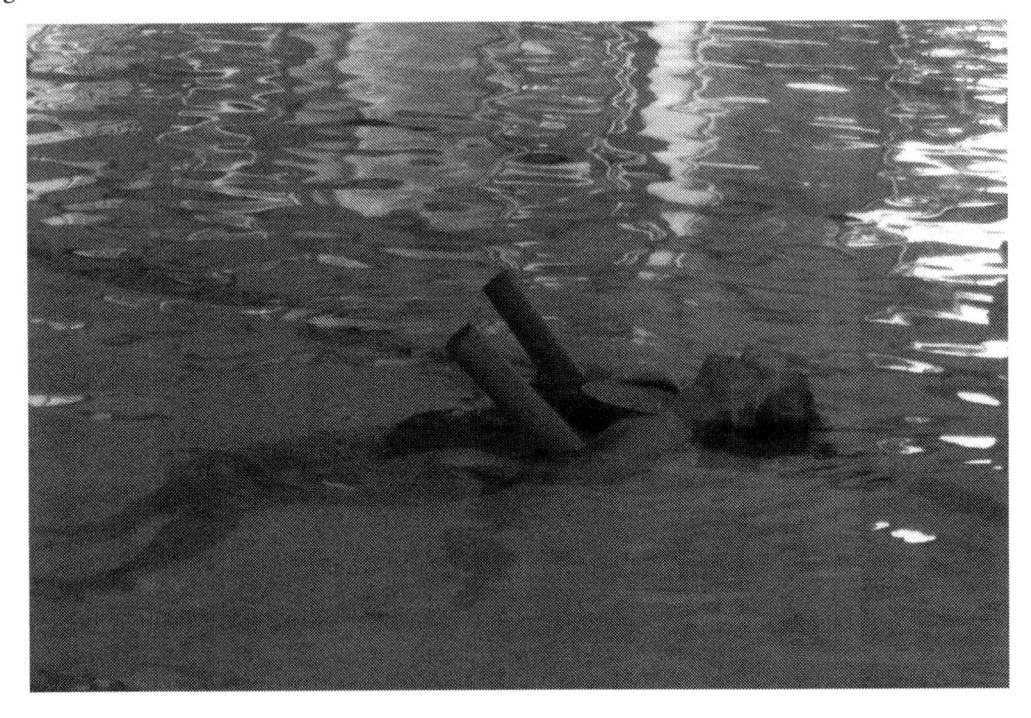

The spanda or vibration under water is more acute than on land. A wonderful way for the experienced yoga student to explore pratyahara (sense withdrawal)

Typical Students

Providing students are healthy and/or have permission from a doctor, the typical group could include the following people:

* Overweight students
* Those with swollen joints
* People who love water exercise generally
* Those with arthritis
* Some wheelchair users (Check if pool chair lift available)
* People with balance issues such as M.S.
* Pre-natal (especially those who are preparing for a water birth)
* Post-natal students
* Older adults
* Those who prefer gentler exercise or are new to exercise
* Those with minimal body awareness
* Those who are on vacation and have access to a pool
* Serious yoga students practicing self-study
* Competitive swim students
* Synchronized swimmers
* Young swimmers
* People curious about yoga, but prefer the water environment
* Those with erratic breathing patterning
* Those with sleep disorders

Inclusion Yoga

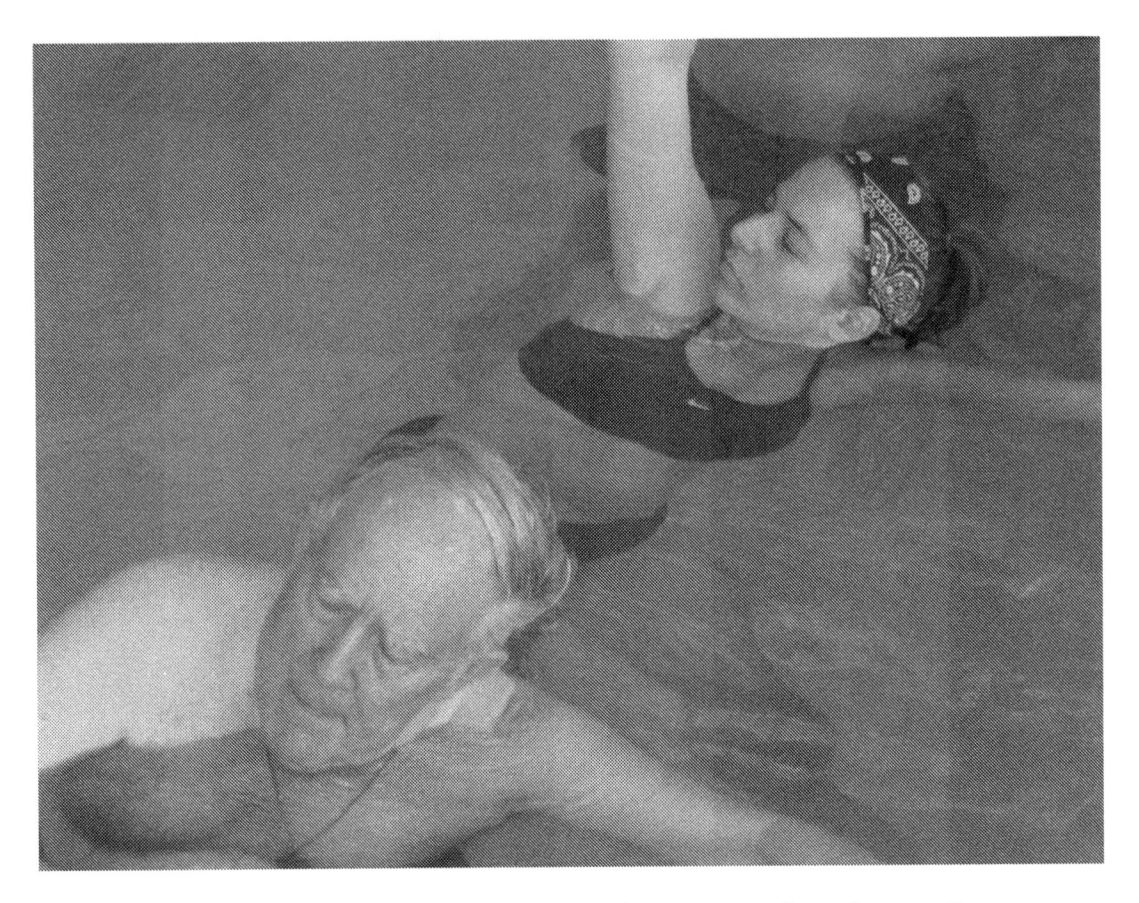

Integration into the class can minimize the sense of separateness from the rest of society.

The wise master said," Seek out your own illumination diligently". In so doing, we should want all souls to be free and able to do the same, in spite of their particular body bias. This bias in the body can give a person a sense of separation from others. Yoga is about us remembering that we are all connected to one another. The only separation is in the mind. Body bias can intensify that feeling of separateness but need not in an inclusion program. The YMCA's in particular are very good in this area.

Asana is only one of the '8 limbs of yoga', that lead to the quieting of the mind stuff and enable us to go deep within to a state of meditation. The journey should be enjoyable.

Whatever reservations I may have had early on in teaching Aqua Yoga have long been eradicated as I keep on hearing the same positive feedback from students who have made exercise in the water a part of their health regime.

The Saratoga YMCA in particular, has a wonderful inclusion program that encourages diversity of abilities in some classes. It teaches all students to become more compassionate and tolerant of other people, regardless of the condition of their body, or handicap.

The breath is the main focus in any yoga class, and really is where most of the work needs to be done to enable us to feel better about ourselves, and radiate that positive energy out to other souls seeking the same. Many self conscious people feel the water to be a safe environment to work on the breath and body, and gain greater confidence and coordination. It gives them a sense of independence and self-esteem, which may be lacking.

Sometimes, students who seem very strong and confident generally can become fearful when it comes to floating at the end of class. I usually get into the water at this time, and encourage these students to try and surrender. They have a foam noodle under their armpits and another one under the knees, and so are nicely cradled between the two. They may still not be ready to 'let go' of course, and that should be their decision and not the teachers. Some comments have included those who feel such a sense of accomplishment, never daring to think they could do that, simply because they have not done it before.

Soft music in the background, and on a sunny day, spotlights of the sun's rays through the skylights, the students find their place in the sun to float, and contemplate the after effects of the class.

Introduction

"As above. So below." Our planet is made up of around 70% water, the same as the human body. We cannot separate ourselves from this medium, and if we open our minds, we can even conceive of taking our self- inquiry, or starting our hatha yoga practice in the water, especially if there is some body bias that needs special attention.

Our current physical and mental limitations can be changed. Take for example, a child's molded creation made from some dough, and re-shape it into something, anything else. Mystically speaking, although our personality is 'baked', we can change our hardened attitudes, by becoming more aware of the subtle aspects that go to make up who we think we are. The greater our self-awareness, the more control we have in our lives.

At first, when I was asked to teach "Aqua Yoga", I was very apprehensive, and even skeptical about its validity. I am, after all, what I consider, a serious yoga student and teacher, trying to 'live my practice.' This self- doubt, I have come to recognize is my ego getting in the way of helping many people find ways of transforming their lives through the practice of yoga.

Yoga is many thousands of years old, and the Yoga Sutras of Patanjali stress that asana practice should be done with "comfort and stability", and no one should judge what, or where another's comfort zone is.

As practitioners of Yoga, it is our dharma, or duty to sow the seeds of conscious action in other people, so that they can improve their lives, wherever they may be on their path, if in fact they want to improve their lives.

As a child, I had joined a synchronize swimming class which I was moderately good at, but foolishly dropped after a few years as interest waned, and mum and dad no longer had the energy to force me to keep going. That experience however is deeply rooted in my memory track, and the experience of this terribly difficult discipline has fuelled my belief that Aqua Yoga is in fact a viable option for all students of yoga who like being in the water. In the right environment, with the right attitude, it is possible to experience the same sense of balanced self-awareness that one can obtain (also with the right attitude) on land.

Ultimately, the student tries to take the practice off of the 'sticky mat', and into their lives, so that whatever we are doing, we are doing so mindfully. One of my dear devoted students listens to one of my asana tapes every night whilst lying in bed after many surgical procedures and suffering with chronic pain, yet still gains meaning, moving the more subtle energies of the body. He visualizes and moves his body in the direction of the pose, which is really following a "Pranic, model" of the asana. The focused breathing helps to keep the mind creative and alert. We can even heighten our awareness of ujjayi (victorious breath) and uddiyana bandha (inner lengthening of subtle and physical bodies) in the water if the student is adept in yoga. Everyone has their own unique timing mechanism, and we have to respect where everyone is on their path.

The breath, as my beautiful Guru says, is the doorway to cosmic consciousness, and we all have to breathe to sustain this earth life. The alchemical process of inner and outer transformation, starts here, and so the breath, like any other hatha class should be the primary focus.

Bridging the Mind and Body

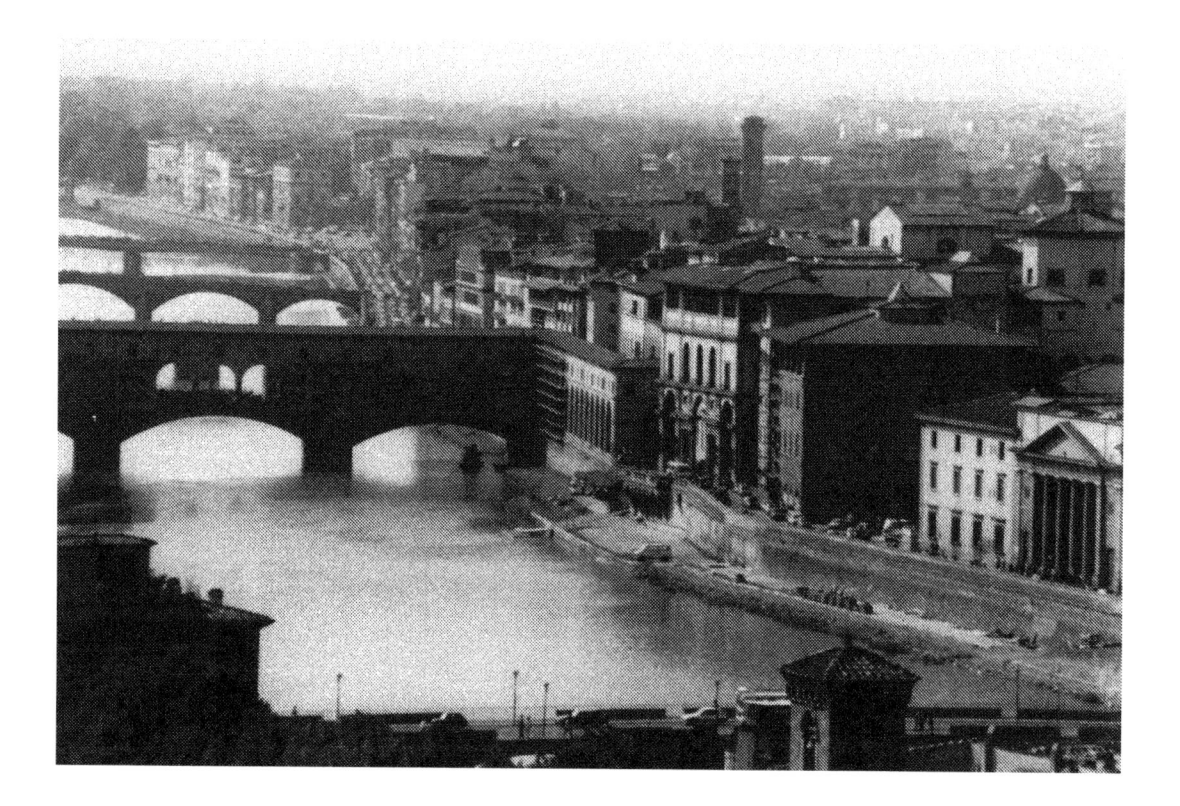

Beautiful Bridges in Florence, Italy.

Hatha yoga is a way to bridge the gap between the mind and body, bringing it to a state of communion, unaffected by emotionality or angular energy. We have allowed our minds to become manipulated by external noises and confusion, which causes us to swing from one state of consciousness to another, and loose the primordial continuity of consciousness that is centered deep within us all. This causes us to become fearful, judgmental and greedy. The body and the mind reflects these traits by its imbalance or bias. The breath and its control can also create a bridge between the body and mind, such that we can become more comfortable in the body, and therefore in the mind.

Yoga is not an easy path to tread. We have to be prepared to 'get our feet wet' symbolically, to create a new flow in our lives that can transform us forever.

As our awareness deepens, we become more aware of the subtle bodies or astral and causal bodies. In the same way, we can look out at the stars and planets in awe, and feel like a very small part of the cosmic wheel of manifestation.

We can start to take charge of our universe, which is our mind and body, because we see that it is only a temporary dwelling place, yet a vehicle to experience something greater than ourselves.

According to Patanjali, we have some obstacles in the mind stuff that need to be removed. They are as follows:

1. Forgetfulness
2. Ego
3. Aversion
4. Attraction
5. Attachment to the physical body

These obstacles are known as Kleshas, and are in the way of us achieving Samadhi. (unification with the Universal Spirit)

Most of the obstacles, by way of prejudice, and loyalty, have been stored in our memory track from many incarnations. These could be universal, cultural or individual. An example my guru uses is a bike. Universally known as a means of transportation. Culturally to the Chinese the main means of getting about, but to an American, mostly something used for exercise and enjoyment. On an individual level, maybe a symbol of joy, or something very scary and dangerous. Unlike the physical body, these memory tracks called samskaras do not die when the physical body dies. They go to make up the law of cause and effect that is known as karma. These prejudices, loyalties and cultural indoctrination's give rise to fluctuations of the mind, known as vrittis. The goal of yoga is to remove these. Most of the problems we face are not "out there", in our family, culture or civilization, but contained within our mind.

A bridge is, "A structure that spans a river, road, or lake." In yoga, the structure is the skeleton. If the bones are in correct alignment, we can open up the joints, lengthen and strengthen the muscle groups, and feel much more comfortable in our body. In conjunction with the comfortable body, it is the breath that needs to be changed in order for us to become more aware of the subtle energies within the subtle bodies. These energies are known as Prana.

Another definition of a bridge is: "A platform that runs from one side of a ship to another that is for the officer in charge." For most of us, we have not become the captain of our inner ship, which has a huge cargo of uncontrolled thoughts. We are not responsible for the thoughts as they have always existed, but we are responsible for what we do with them, and how we let them affect us and other people.

"The Ego is like a stick dividing water into two.
It creates the impression that you are one and
I am another. When the ego vanishes you will
Realize that Brahman is your own inner consciousness"

Ramakrishna - "The Wisdom of the Hindu Gurus" by Timothy Freke

The Lotus as a Metaphor in Yoga

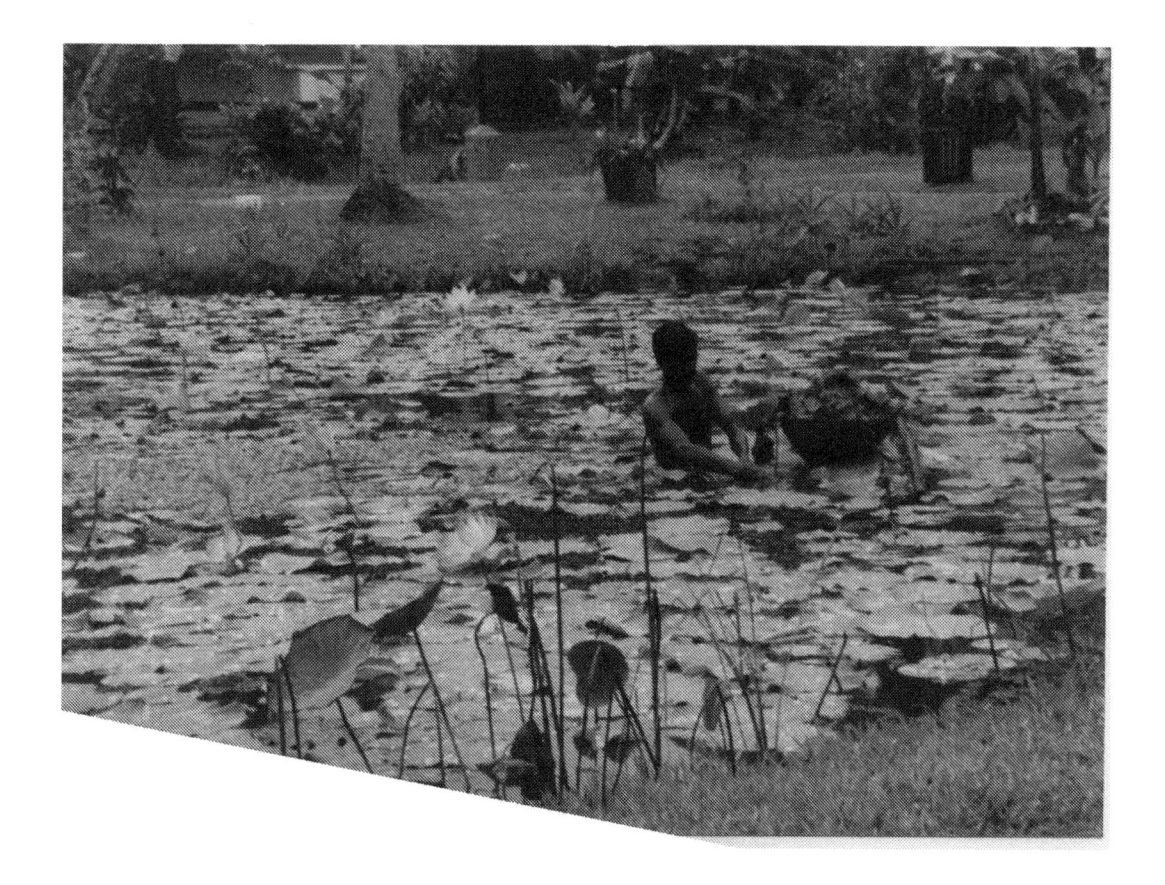

I took this photograph at an Ayurvedic center in Kerala, South India. The lotus is often used as a symbol in yoga as a metaphor for spiritual evolution. A symbol of detachment.

Here, the worker is thinning out the weeds deep in the murky depths of the pond. The beautiful lotus has a rather ugly and large, very tangled root system that needs to be trimmed every so often. Rather like the thoughts in the mind. My guru uses the acronym SPOT. First you have to spot the problems, then prioritize them, organize and then trim them.

Yoga is an inner alchemy as much as it is an external one. Its effects are more lasting however because they are not limited by the physical body.

"THE WORLD IS IN ANGUISH BECAUSE THE MINDS OF MEN ARE IN ANGUISH."

SHELLY - Kriya Lineage

The Churning of the Mind stuff

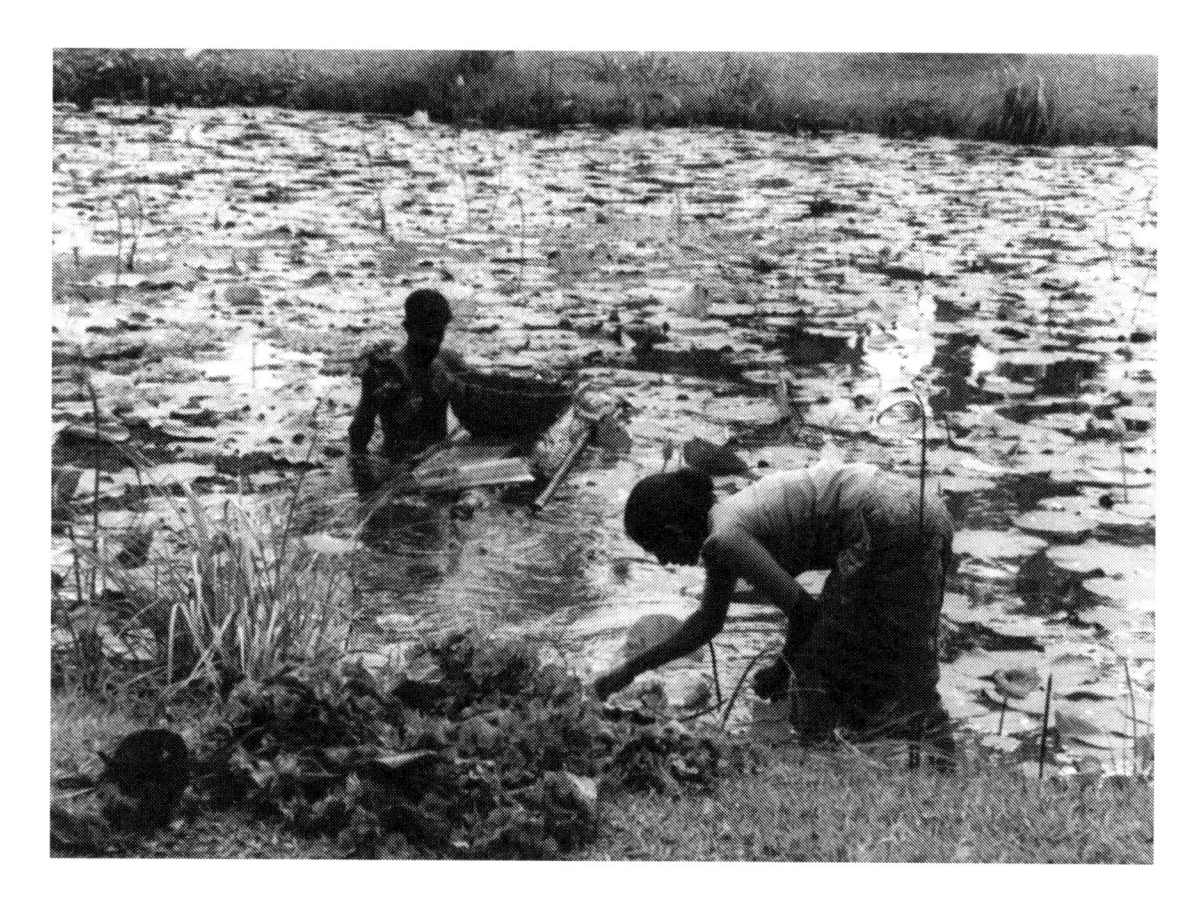

   Once upon a yogi time, there was a Raj who lost a beautiful gem in a large, muddy pond. He asked a passing yogi to perform a special puja and help his servants know where to find it. The yogi sat in posture and focused at the point between his eyebrows, and then proceeded to sit, and sit and sit. The Raj was in continual rage, ranting and raging and eventually demanded that the yogi do something quickly lest his gem be lost forever. The yogi nodded and then pointed at the pond. "See, now we have waited for the churned muddy waters to clam down, we can see clearly into the pond and find your treasure".

   We are mystically, the beautiful lotus that appears to just float on the surface of the water, yet has it roots deep below in the mud. Just like the gardener that was thinning out the weeds in the photograph of the pond, we have to thin out the thoughts in our mind to a manageable quantity. The next step is to categorize them and discern what is right or wrong knowledge, a memory, or the product of a vivid imagination. This takes constant and continual practice and dispassion as outline in Patanjali's Yoga Sutras, to see ourselves as we really are. The lovely lotus. Ultimately, yoga is about getting rid of 'stuff, and not 'getting' anything. Life should become simpler and less complicated, not more so.

   We have, as humans, come a long way from the 'cave of the ancient
   yogis', and are bombarded with radio's, televisions and noisy people generally.

A particular sound can trigger a certain memory that manifests in a habitual reaction patterning. These patterns get churned up whenever a trigger that causes us emotionality is set. For some, it is a dog barking. For some a child crying. Whatever the agitation is, we need to break free from destructive thoughts as they get churned up by events, people or places.

There are some floatation tanks that contain water of exactly the same temperature as the human body. The chamber is dark, and it takes a very short time to drift into a sleep state here because we have no awareness of the senses. In prison, the worst punishment for most offenders, would be to put them into solitary confinement because they are left alone with the churning thoughts in their mind. Much easier perhaps to be in a noisy environment, where we can forget the Mind stuff altogether ,or simply blackout and fall asleep rapidly.

This is forgetfulness however and the result, of delusion often known as maya, or the veiling principle. This is mistaking the impermanent for permanent. All is change. What we want today, we get tomorrow, but when tomorrow comes, we tend to want something else. This is man's dilemma and causes us much suffering.

"AND NEAR HIM STOOD THE LADY OF THE LAKE, WHO KNOWS A SUBTLER MAGIC THAN HIS OWN -CLOTHED IN WHITE SAMITE, MYSTIC, WONDERFUL, SHE GAVE THE KING HIS HUGE CROSSHILTED SWORD".

Alfred Tennyson - The coming of Arthur

<u>Connecting to the Inner Mermaid</u>

I have long since been fascinated by myths and stories of mermaids, like the Lady of the Lake rising from the misty lake at Avalon, and as a child remember a favorite birthday card that had a lovely mermaid on the front combing her golden locks.

Very often, they can be depicted as naughty and seductive, but there is something mystically magnetic about a living being that is neither of just the land, or just the water. Maybe in the future, we could find ourselves living in 'Atlantis' . We seem so intent on destroying the land we already have.

The mermaid is seen on a rock, gazing out to sea, as a haunting vibration fills the air. The Irish name for mermaid means 'song of the sea', or sea chant. She is often sitting in an oyster shell, a string of pearls for her mala. For centuries, people believed that pearls were formed by a drop of rain falling into an open oyster where upon it immediately congealed into a pearl. Many legends and poems were based around this theory.

"And precious the tear, as the rain from the sky, which turns into pearl as it flows in the sea."

'Errors, like straws upon the surface flow;
He who would search For pearls must dive below'

'God's Jewels - Their Dignity and Destiny' W.Y. Fullerton

Swiss Knight, Ulrich Von Zatzikhoven in the twelfth century claims that, the mermaid or Queen of Maidenland, in his text Lanzelot, is none other than the Lady of the Lake in the Arthurian legend.

Listening to the music as the waves pound the beaches is very relaxing, and for this reason, many people love to relax by the water. It could be on a beach somewhere, or by a lake or river, but even a bubbly bath can be a therapeutic haven.
There is something quite nurturing about floating in the water. It allows us to offer less resistance and go with the flow of life. We just have to remember that we are self-existent beings. If I can think a thought, I can become it. We can break free from our emotional suffering, and find a happier place to dwell deep within ourselves.

ESTABLISHING THE BREATH IN MOUNTAIN POSE

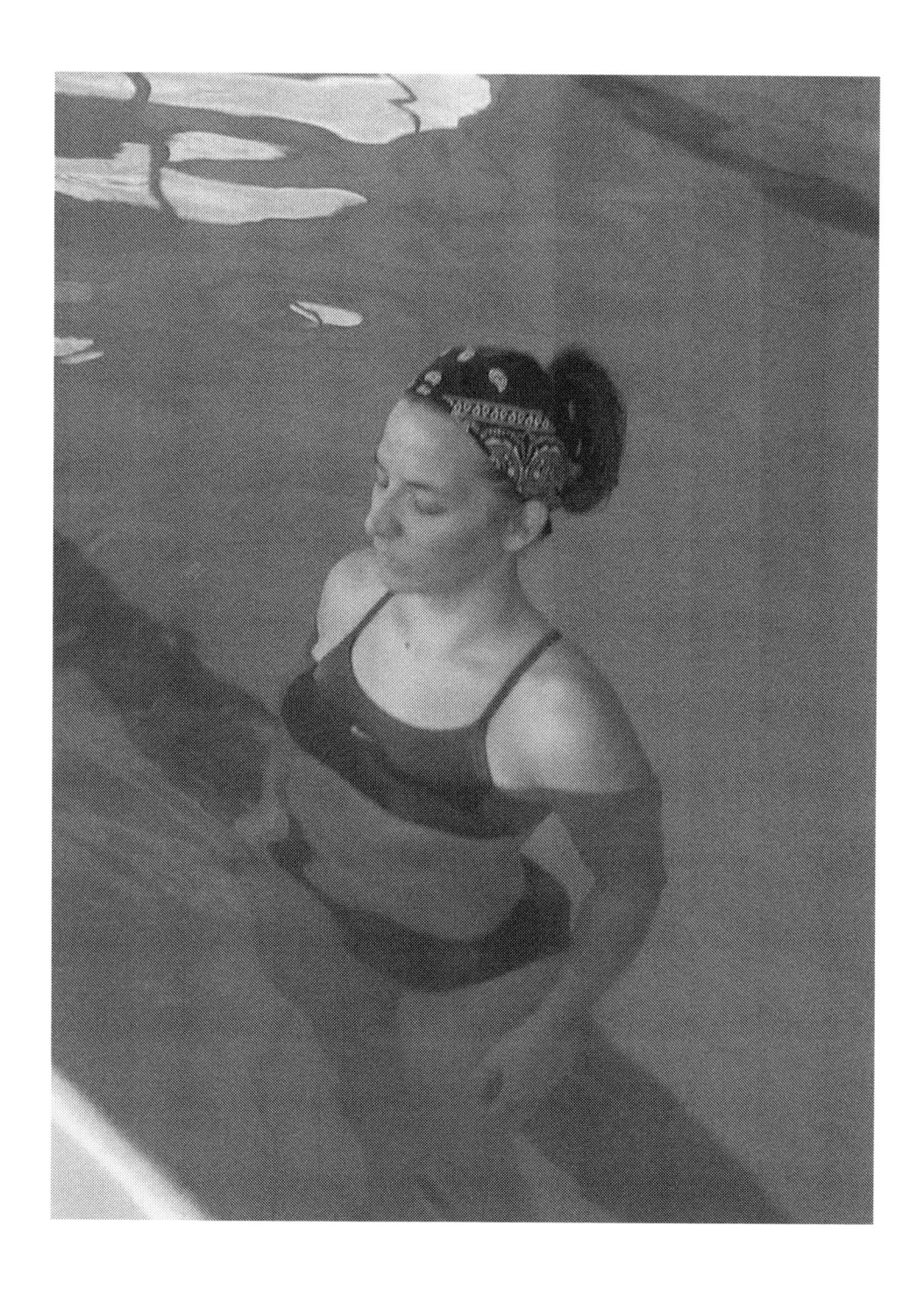

The Breath

The first thing I get my students to do, is line up along the edge of the pool and ask them to tell me, "What are we all doing here?" They reply, "Breathing".

A silly ritual perhaps, but nonetheless, one that starts us off on the right footing. It helps the students to remember to focus, and me to prepare for presenting the teachings to a class of students who may be in kindergarten in terms of body and mind awareness. I usually get them to close their eyes as they stand strong in mountain pose, and chant, "inhale, exhale," a few times to help find a common thread. This ritual is repeated at the end of the class before they float in corpse or floating savasana. Actually some joke that they only breathe on Friday and would like to see that on a bumper sticker.

Here, in Mountain pose, the students can practice how to breathe from the belly, to the back and then to the space under the collarbones on an inhale and then back down the trunk through the exhale. The belly moves out on the inhale and back to the spine through the exhale.)

This quiet time can be useful to the teacher also to see who has good posture, or who may show some real bias. She can also see who may need to move into deeper or more shallow water. Water about chest level could be about right for most of the work. Go too deep and they cannot bend their knees without taking their head under water. Experience will lead the student to their preferred depth of water.

Many of the students feel much better after one class because they breathe in a different way to how the body has become habituated. One lovely large student told me about a time when she was sitting in the park practicing her breathing, when a stranger came up to her and commented on her composure and serenity. No one had complimented her on her physical appearance for many years, and this was an enormous boost for her self- confidence.

This is so indicative of how it is in yoga. Many people around us notice positive changes in us before we notice them ourselves.

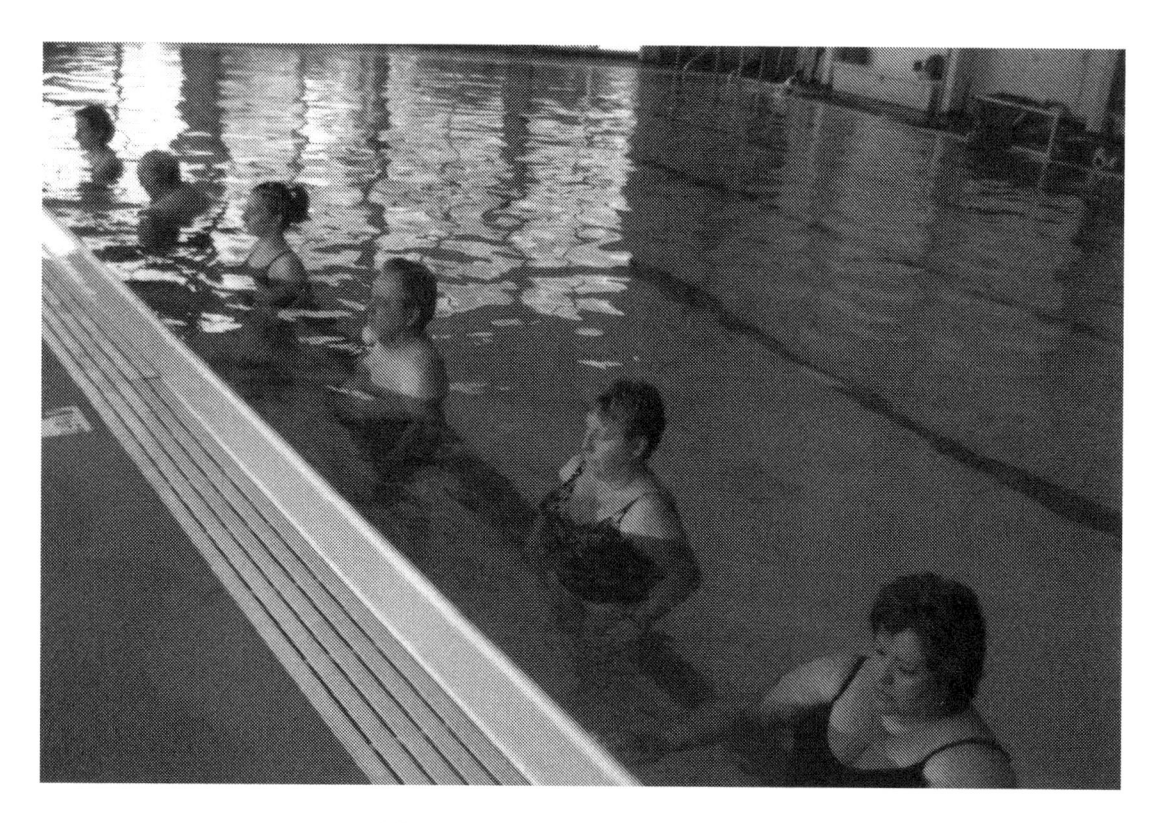

ATTUNING TO STILLNESS AS A GROUP

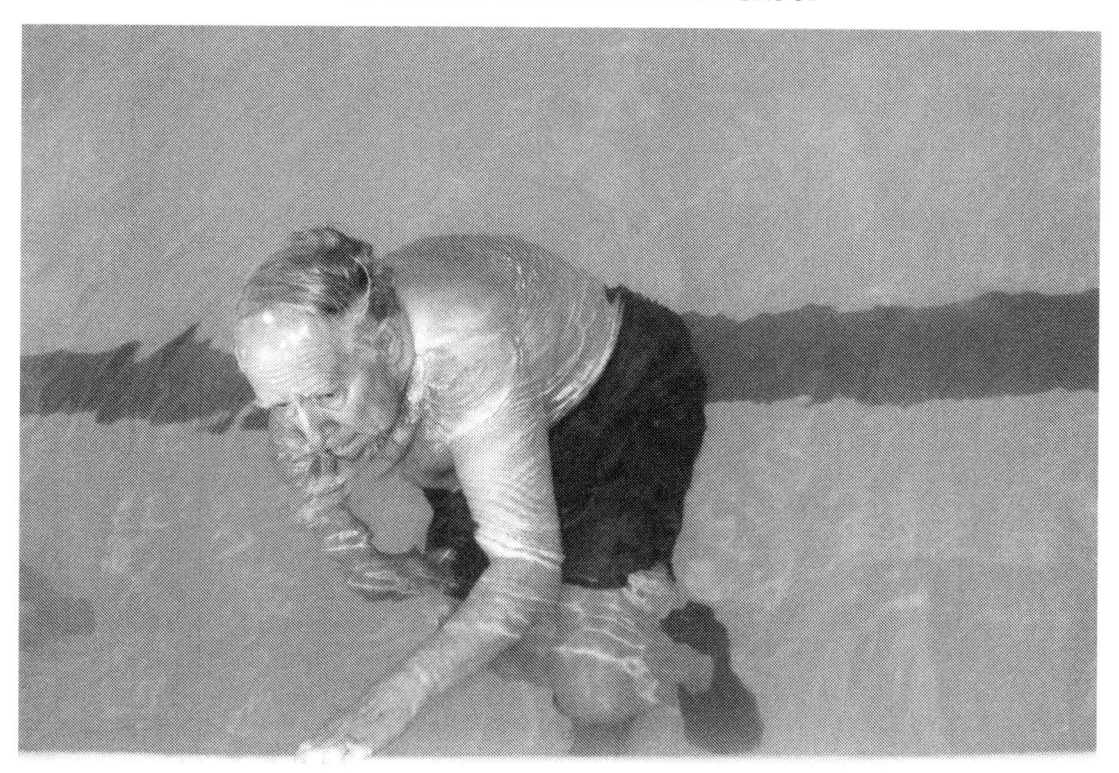

STROKE SURVIVORS CAN FIND MEANING IN CLASS TOO

The Pool Requirements

Just as we like to create a yoga studio with an amiable ambiance for the students to practice in on land, so too should we strive to create the same nurturing atmosphere in the pool area. Here are some guidelines;

* Pool temperature should be a minimum of 84 degrees, ideally higher. Adapted 'sun salutations' or 'walking warrior' can help here if the pool feels chilly.

* Students should be able to stand at the side of the pool in chest high water. It is my belief that using the side of the wall as a prop in Aqua Yoga affords better articulation of the asanas, and also allows the teacher better access to assisting the student. (This as opposed to asana practice away from the wall)

* No drafts if an indoor pool.

* Nobody splashing around in the pool area at the same time which can be very distracting to the class environment. Understanding and cooperation from the organization offering the class is needed here.

* In a class setting the teacher must be heard, so check out the acoustics. Some teachers may need to use a microphone, or it's a great chance to practice voice projection.

* About 1 hr is probably enough for both teacher and student.

* Music at the end can help students stay focused and minimize the need to talk. Simply relax in adapted savasana. (floating corpse)

* In class setting a lifeguard and /or caregiver should be at hand.

* Props can include foam noodles, kick boards and dumb bells.

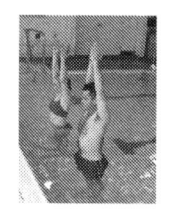

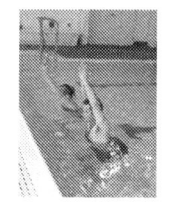

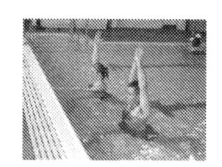

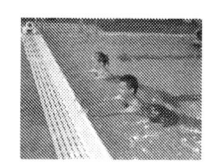

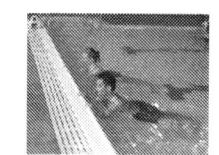

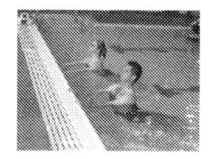

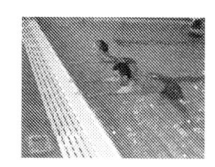

The Sequencing of Asanas

Time, Place and Circumstance affects the way in which we need to approach life, and the teacher or student has to be comfortable in the medium of water in the same way that they need to be comfortable on land. The water may be cooler than desirable sometimes. The students may have a short attention span and the cool water and lack of self awareness in the group, like on land would determine how best to structure and pace the class.

Repetition of asanas can be good at helping the students gain attention and an awareness of the body. They can then become more aware of the breath and where they need to refine that.

Goswami Kriyananda refers to Tadasana or Mountain Pose as the Maha asana, or the great asana. He refers to the concept of being able to stand on our own two feet. This is not a physical concept but a mental one, where we don't expect anyone else to sort our problems out. We alone can create, sustain and dissolve our inner universe. In so doing, we can have an affect on the outer one. On a physical level, some students may be used to sitting in a wheel chair all day, and the buoyancy in the water can give them a real boost psychologically because they may find they can stand on their own two feet with the help of the pool wall.

I find that some movement across the width of the pool, in walking warrior for example, can increase the cardiovascular element of the class, which can be necessary if the student is feeling cool. If they are easily distracted, and or lack discipline, it can also create a focus for their scattered mind.

The overall effect of the class should allow the student to feel more relaxed and balanced. It should incorporate hip and shoulder openers, as well as spine extension, flexion, lateral bends and twists, (students may have bias, so may not be appropriate for all of them)

I may start the class off with small movements like turning head from side to side, chin to chest, head back, and then move on to shoulder rotations, hip circles and so on, before moving on with some of the more classical poses. Breaking the asanas or postures down into easily understood components is necessary before stringing them together as a flow, or vinyassa. Paying attention to how well the student is listening and interpreting what the teacher is saying along with how they are breathing should determine how the class develops, rather than having a fixed agenda.

A while ago, I had a student tell me that she had pushed herself very hard for many years as a "lap swimmer", and could not believe how intense yoga is, and the enormous positive effect it had on her.

Self- awareness is not easy, and breathing and thinking correctly is not an easy option for those who find it difficult to motivate themselves to exercise. The mind though can be trained to become stronger, just as we can train the body, and this combination can have a startling effect in our overall sense of well being.

Let the breath awareness develop, and take the asana sequence from that point of origin. There is no destination as such, just a journey that is unique for each student.

Triangle pose

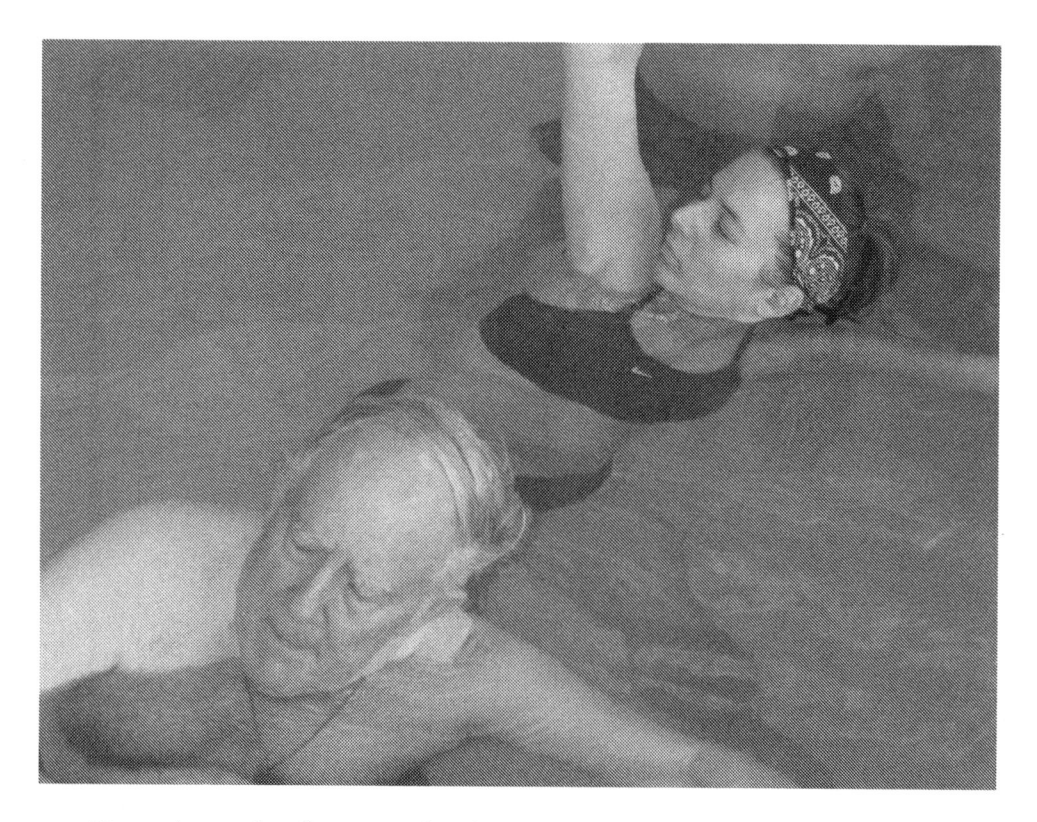

Using the pool wall to articulate better openings of joints and for stability.

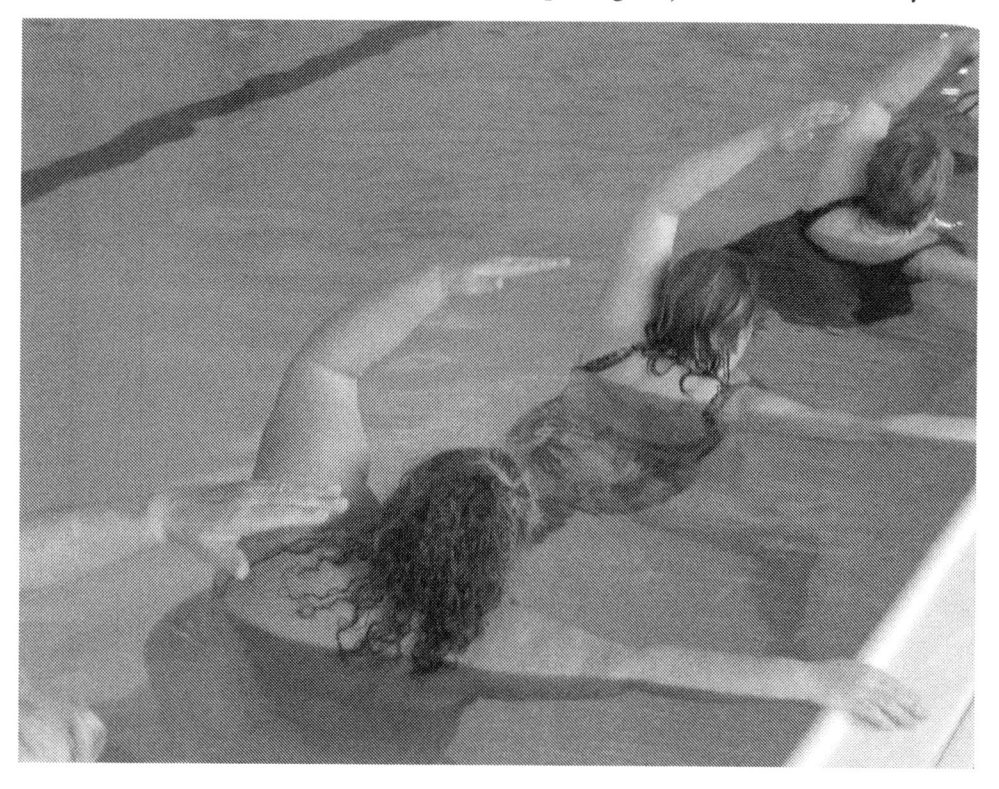

Finding balance in Tree pose

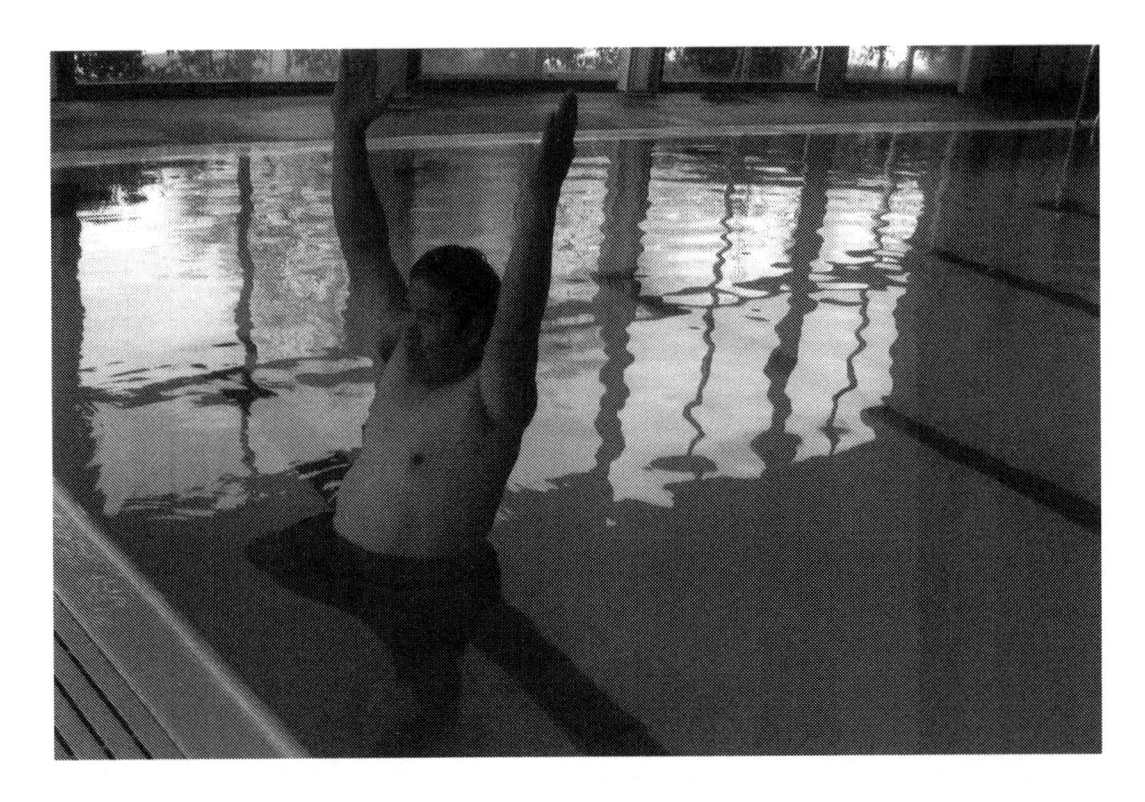

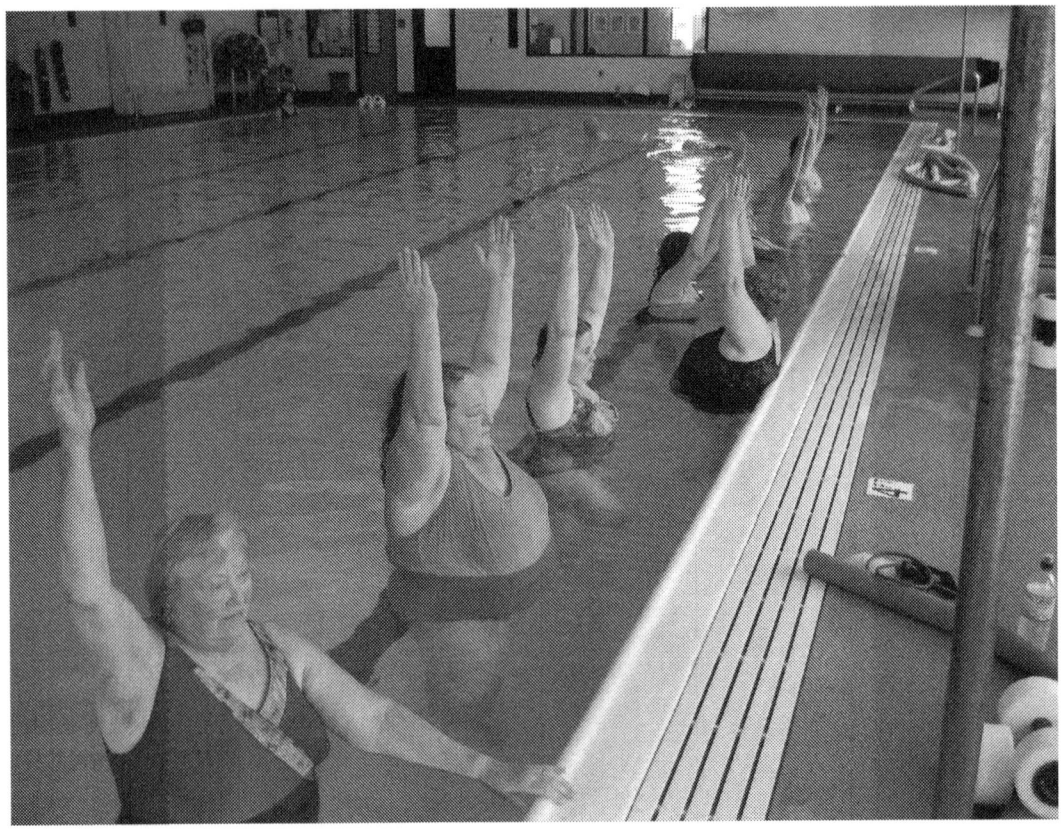

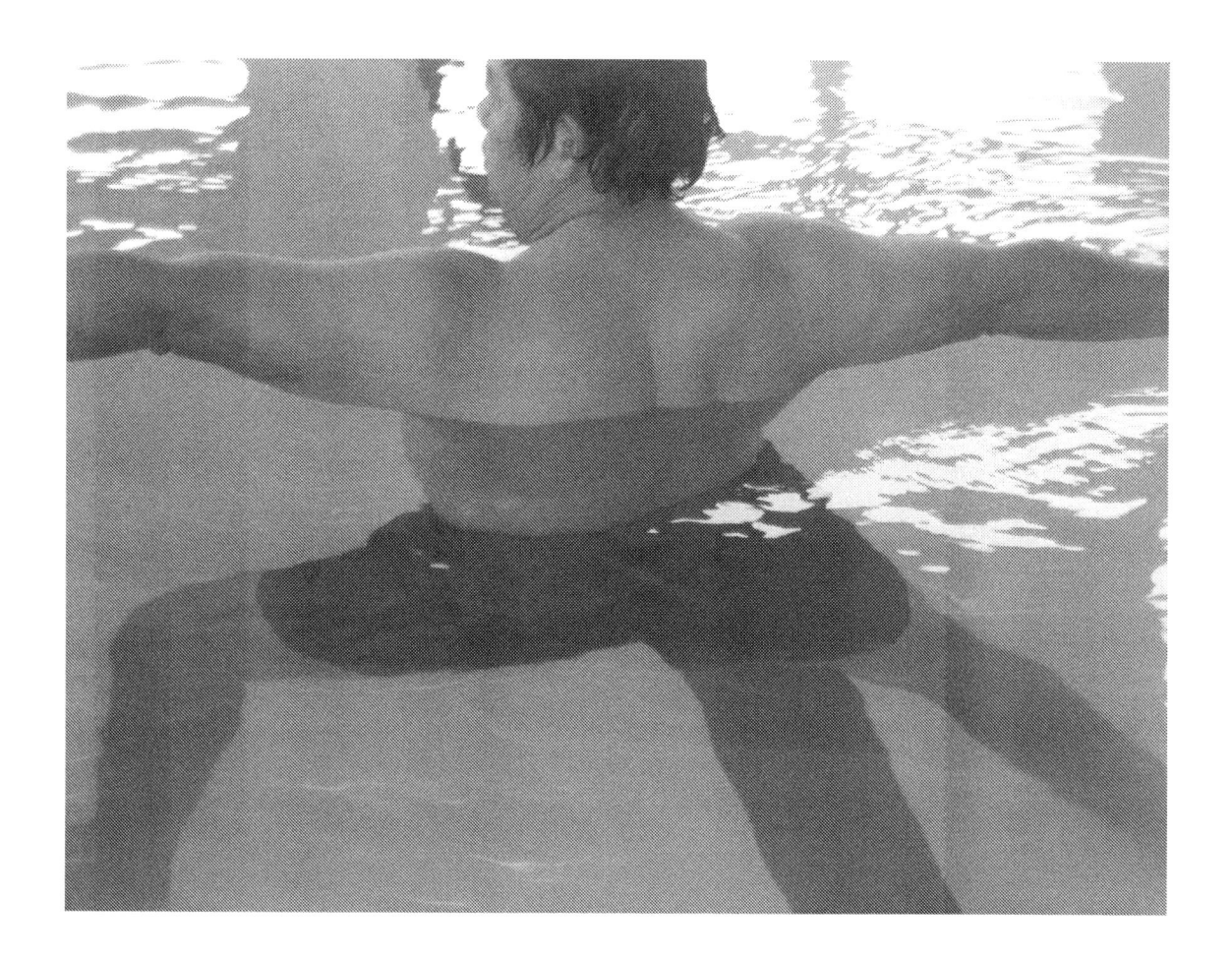

Aqua Yoga and the Competitive Swimmer

Just like we have people coming to yoga classes on land to "cross train", in order to persue their passion, so too can the competitive swimmer, or polo player, or synchronized swimmer, find benefit in practicing Aqua Yoga. As with many intense disciplines, bias can be cultivated in the body with the repetitive training they have to undergo in order to become good at their sport. Cyclists often have hunchbacks and tight hamstrings. They may not want to attend a land class but might find meaning in practicing in the water. The swimmer who only practices front crawl may have tight hips, or may need to refine their breathing patterning. Most people can find some benefits. The synchronized swimmer can enjoy breathing in and out through the nose, and staying longer in the poses generally.

Students can also consider taking some form of yoga class on land, such as restorative, or a beginner's, or an intermediate level class, depending on what is appropriate for them. There are also many chair yoga classes now available, especially in senior centers, YMCA's or community centers. The more the student understands about yoga, the more they will get out of the practice.

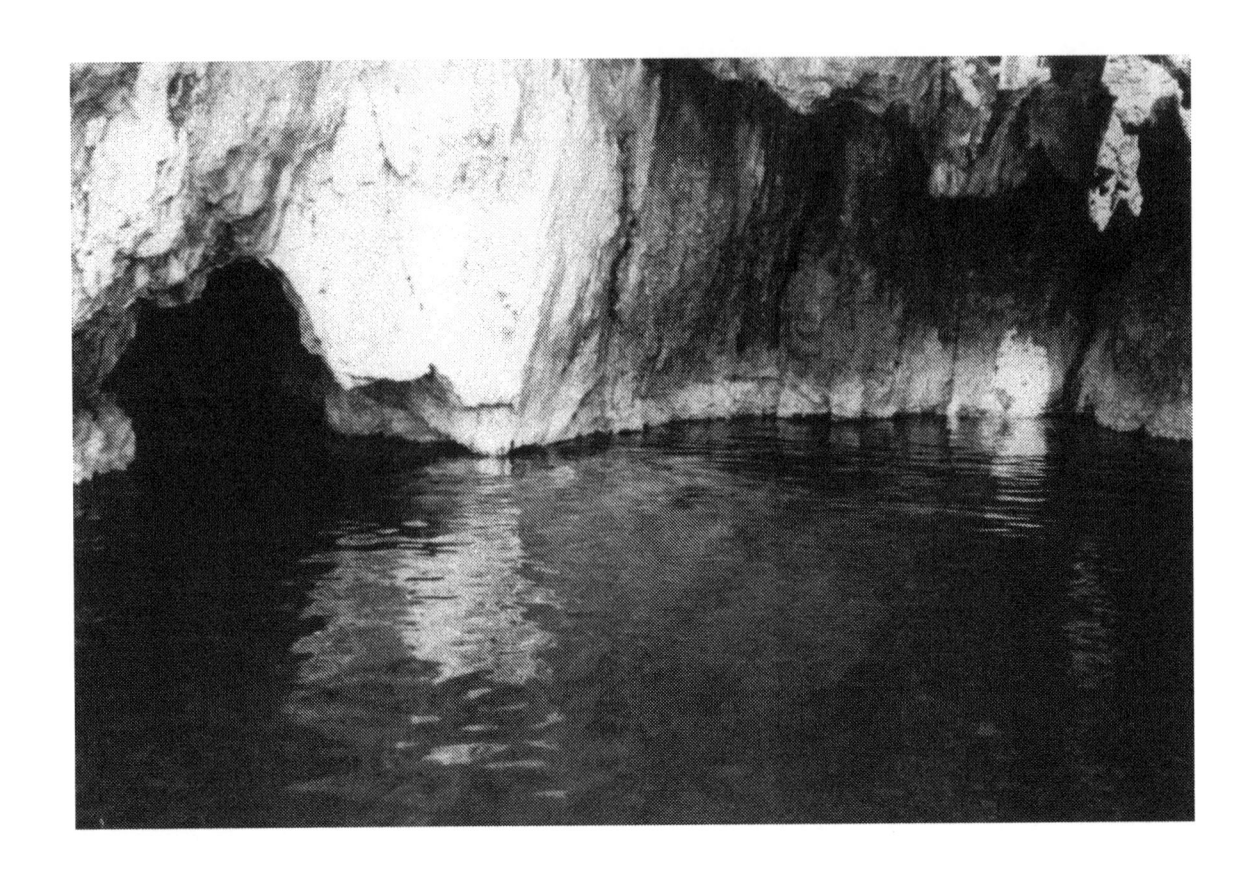

"THIS PERILOUS LIFE IS A DROP OF WATER, A HANGING RAINDROP ON A LOTUS LEAF; SOON IT FALLS BACK IN THE POND BELOW AND IS LOST."

RAMAYANA - William Buck

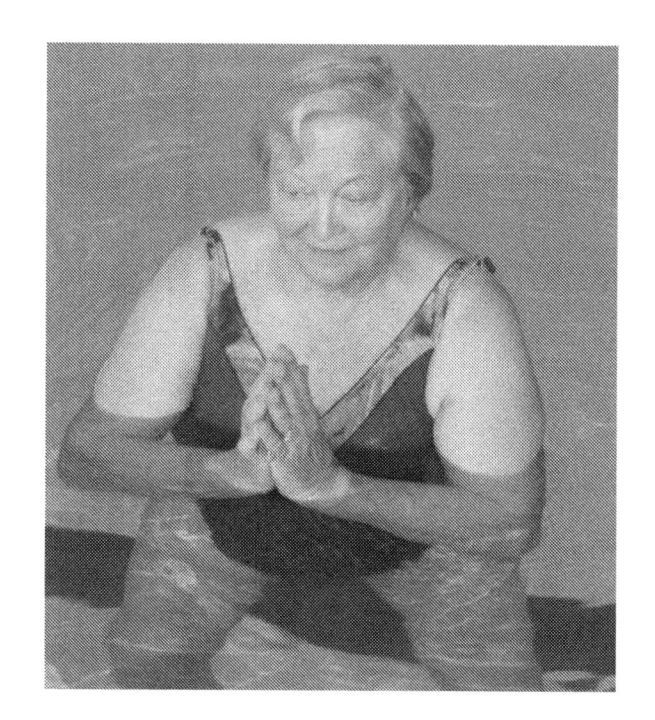

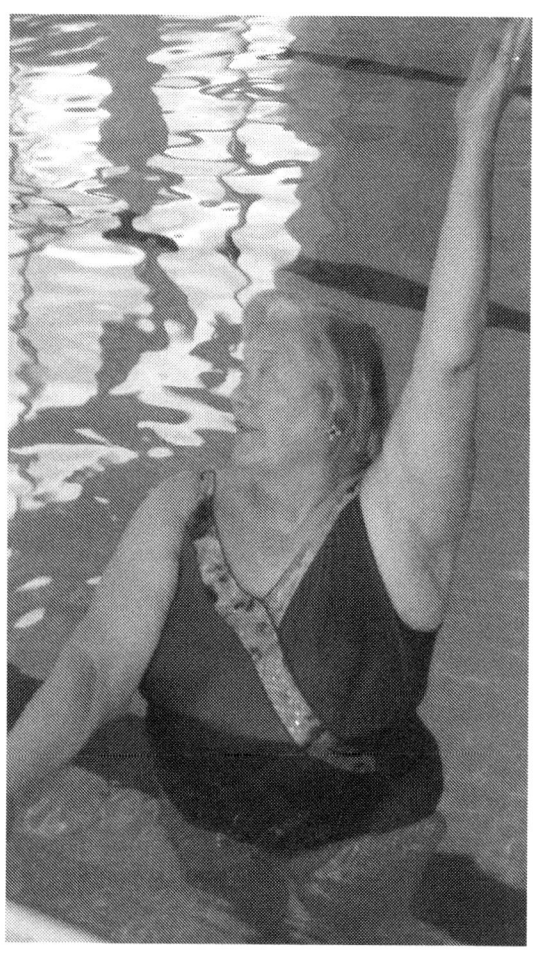

THE ASANAS

(Flowing like a dream, absorbed in the moment I can momentarily feel free to choose)

Aham Brahmasmi -1 am the creative principle....for me.

Tat Twam Asi - That Thou Art

The Asanas

Key Student Instructions

If you are an instructor, or one training to become one, this set of instructions gives you some areas of direction to help lead the students into the asanas, and also some additional refinements to the pose. Most important is that it is fun and that the directions can be heard.

If you are a student and keen to get started yourself, this section will help you. Try not to be too zealous working your way through all asanas in one go with no self- reflection. It is best to try a few in one session and become aware of the effect it is having on your breath and your mind as well as the body. Try to keep focused and not let the mind wander and you will gain much more self- knowledge and contentment with the work you are doing.

Poolside Teacher Notes

Being at the poolside is more effective for the teacher than being in the pool because you can demonstrate clearly what you want them to do. If the student has little body awareness, they may even get confused with a simple instruction like, "Raise your right arm". Using a combination of facing them, and away from them to demonstrate the asanas, gives them an opportunity to understand what, and why you are inviting them to do something, because they can see it clearly for themselves. Being higher up on the deck or poolside, you get a bird's eye view of what they are doing and where they are finding the challenge. Because they are not loading the leg bones in the same way in the externally rotated standing warriors, you can gently assist them move as best as they can without hurting themselves, yet still get a nice hip opener. (A pole or pool net comes in handy here for me, as I sometimes gently touch the inside of a student's knee to help them understand the direction of the thigh bone) Challenged students, for example with a hip replacement seem to do well understanding how to modify the postures for themselves in the water. The water in general I think, is a great place for them to understand skeletal alignment without straining and holding the breath, even though on land it may be a real challenge for them.

Work in the Asanas & Variations

There are many ways of deepening or varying the work, in terms of class content, focus, and direction for all levels of students. The many variations can help to make the class rewarding, even though it may be filled with students who all have different body bias. They are able to work in the direction of the class, even though they may not be doing exactly the same thing as the person standing next to them. This again can give them some inspiration and aspiration to improve the condition of their physical body. This can give them an overall good feeling at the end of the class as they feel they are achieving some mastery over the body and their negativity about what they can, and can't do.

Asana practice and the life Divine

Hatha yoga, or postures and breath/prana (life energies) exercises, are often regarded by Westerners in particular as being yoga, yet is really only the appetizer for the entire menu of yoga, which is a fully integrated system, and considered a sacred science. You do something and it has an effect which is tangible. Yoga, or yoking which is its verb, is a metaphor for the life Divine. A recognition of oneself as part of the greater cosmos, rather that being separate from it, necessitates enjoying one's life to the full and being content. It is essential therefore for each, and every student to feel comfortable with their practice. If possible, they can be encouraged to try some breath work at home and there are many books available on that. Donna Farhi's book on breathing is one that comes for mind.

The breath work and opening up the body, is a superb way to connect with one's higher self.

The Teacher/Student dynamic in Aqua Yoga

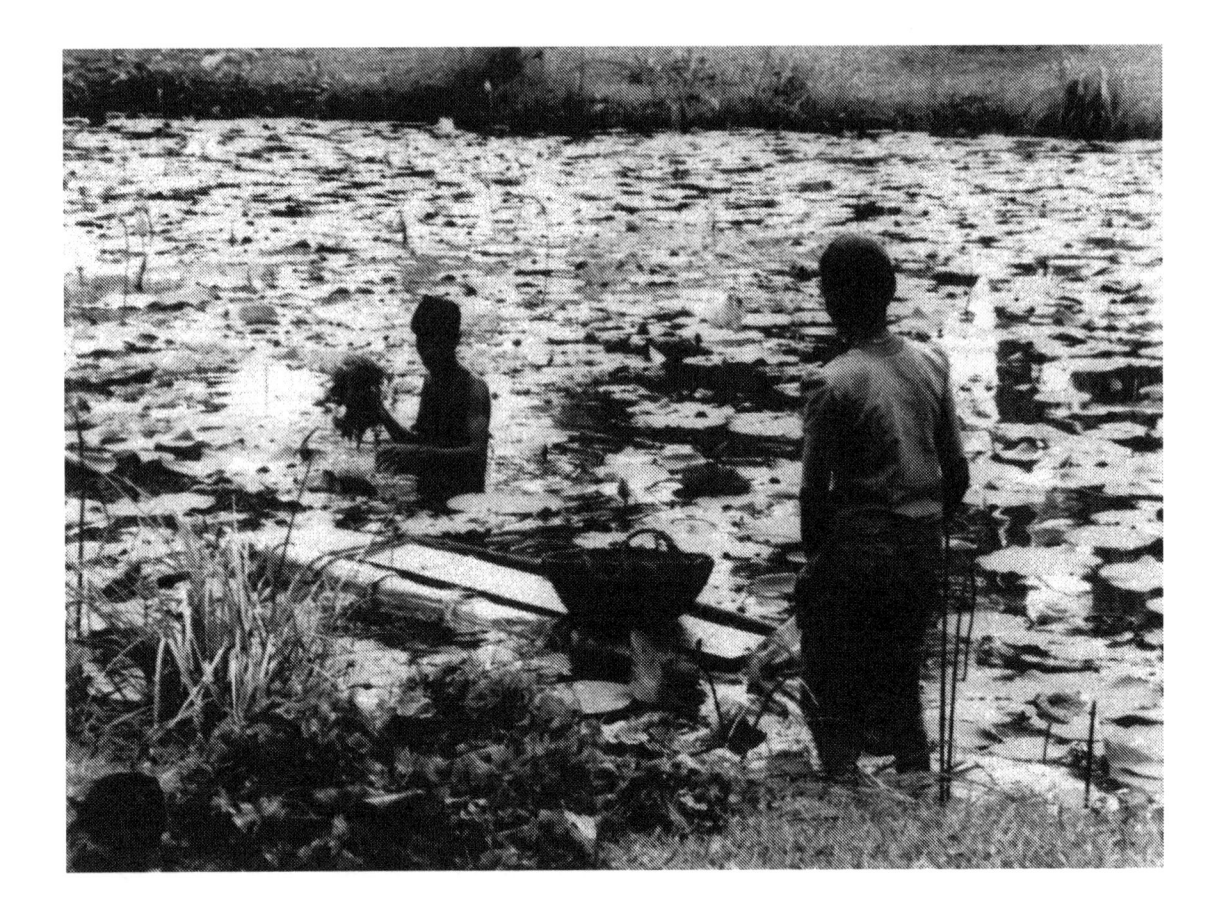

The man in the photograph may loose his awareness of where he is in the pond. She can help him by directing him to a new area, hopefully empowering him to become more proficient with his task. The student, even if just practicing for fun, as a minimum, can expect to be doing some good for the physical body. Communication skills can be worked on in the 'teacher/student' relationship at any level of understanding. When the time is right, more expert guidance can be obtained.

For beginners especially, it is recommended that you seek a class guided by a professional, if not in the water, then, on land, to grasp the fundamentals. Yoga asanas can be very powerful in the fact that they can transform the vehicle of the physical body, but need to be treated with the greatest respect.

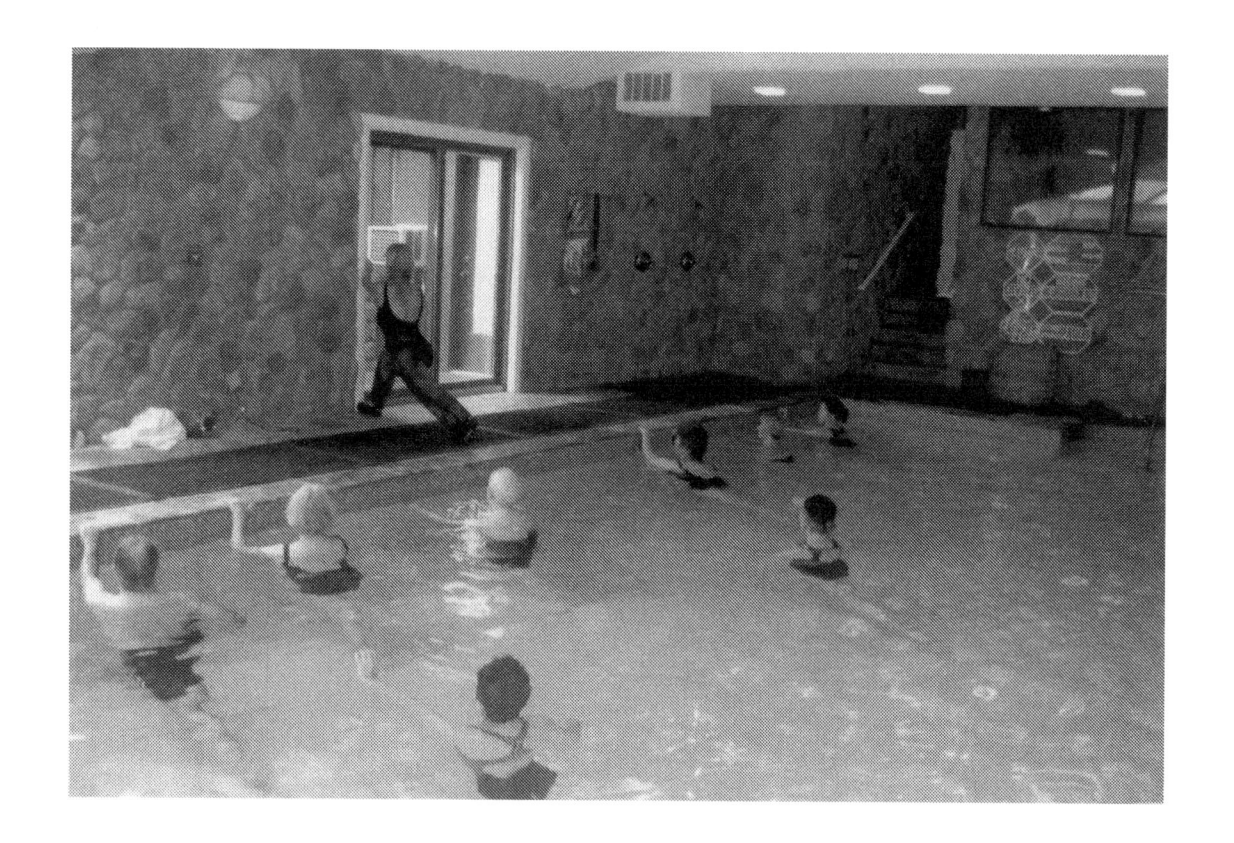

Students with little body awareness and coordination benefit from
the teacher showing them how to organize the body from many angles.

ASANAS – POSTURES

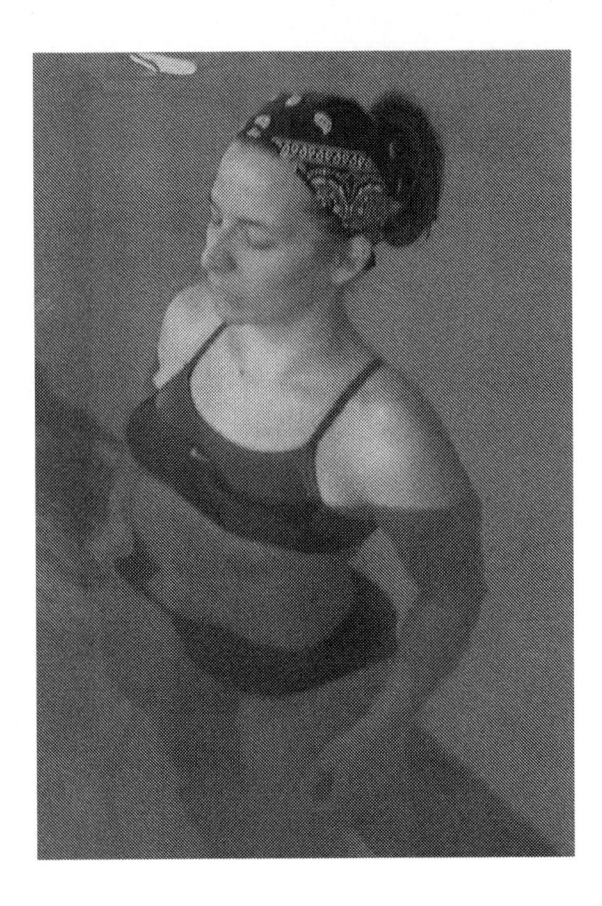

1- MOUNTAIN POSE

KEY STUDENT INSTRUCTIONS

-Stand with feet hip distance toes facing the pool wall.
-Palms by your side.

POOLSIDE TEACHER NOTES

-Check heels apart
-Chin parallel to water surface
-Breathing filling inner walls of the rib cage

Work in Asana or Variations:

-Turn head to right and left. Breathe.
-Shoulder shrugs
-Cross right arm over left, bend elbows and interlace fingers (eagle arms).
-Rotation clockwise and anticlockwise from right hip socket and repeat to left side.
-Cow's face arms (see photo)

1A – Cow's Face Arms

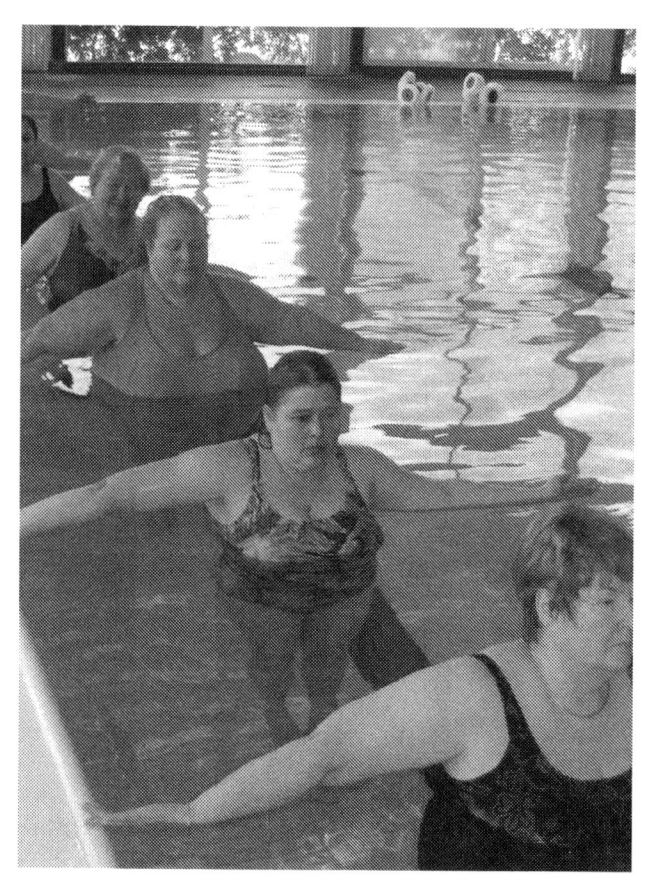

KEY STUDENT INSTRUCTIONS

-Right hand on side on pool deck.
-Internally rotate Right shoulder
-Now, back Right hand to deck.

-Bend Right elbow and try to get back hand between shoulder blades.
-Take Left arm overhead, bend elbow and try to connect hands. Lift heart.

-Repeat other side.

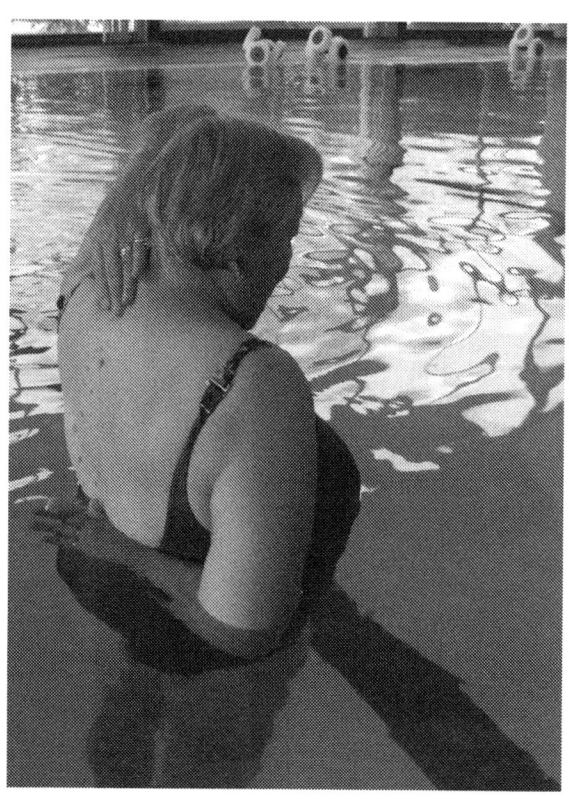

2- Cat – Cow

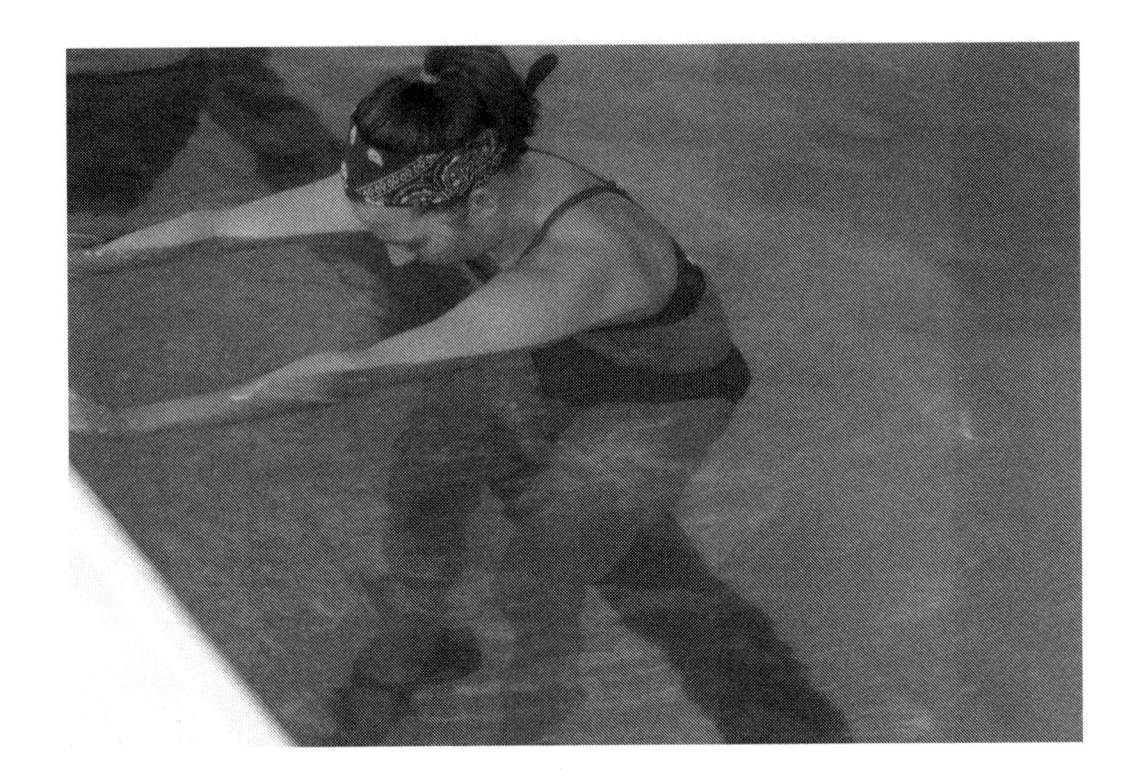

KEY STUDENT INSTRUCTIONS

-Feet hip width distance apart, toes facing the wall.
-Tuck tailbone under and chin down, arching the back (cat pose).
-Rotate pelvis over thighs and deepen the groins, lifting tail bone and looking up (cow pose)

POOLSIDE TEACHER NOTES

-Check coordination
-Exhale to cat.
-Inhale to cow.
-Observe ease or difficulty in this flow.
-It is a good indicator of body biases.

3- Knee to Chest – Leg Stretch

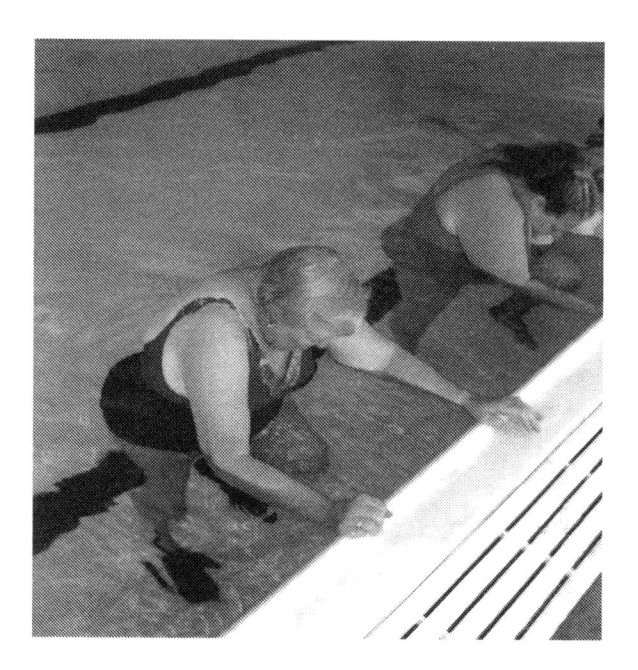

KEY STUDENT INSTRUCTIONS

-Hands to pool deck
-Feet hip width distance
-Exhale right knee to chest
-Inhale extend the right leg behind and toes pointing down.
-Repeat five to 7 times
-Hold pose and keep breathing
-Repeat to the left side

POOLSIDE TEACHER NOTES

-Wrists shoulder width apart
-Tuck chin in
-Toes and knees pointing to the floor and push out through the heel
-Lift the heart

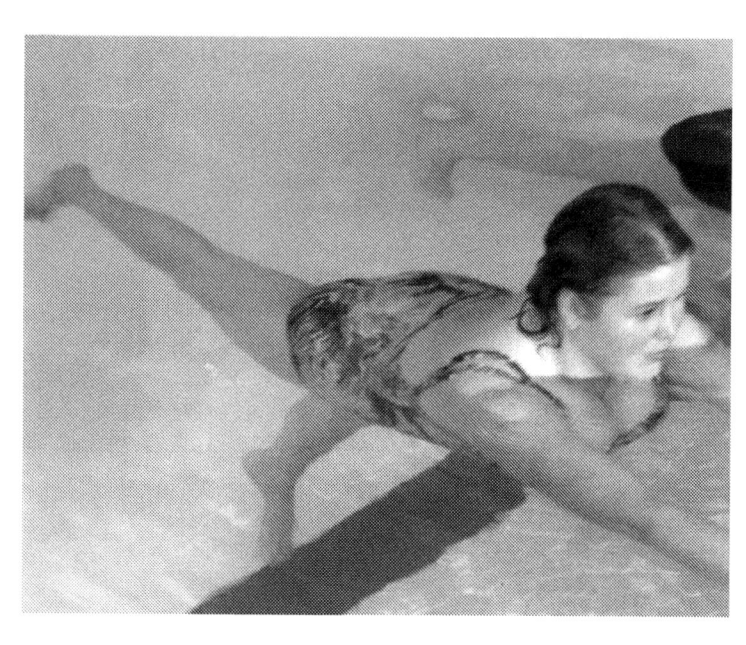

Work in Asana or Variations:

-Stand close to the pool wall
-Bring shin to the wall
-Lift side of the body and extend arms on pool deck.
-Deepen the groins
-Keep shoulders down and armpits deep with strong supported leg.
-**Dancer pose** from mountain
-Reach back and hold the right foot.
-If balance o.k. extend left arm overhead breathing into the back of the body.

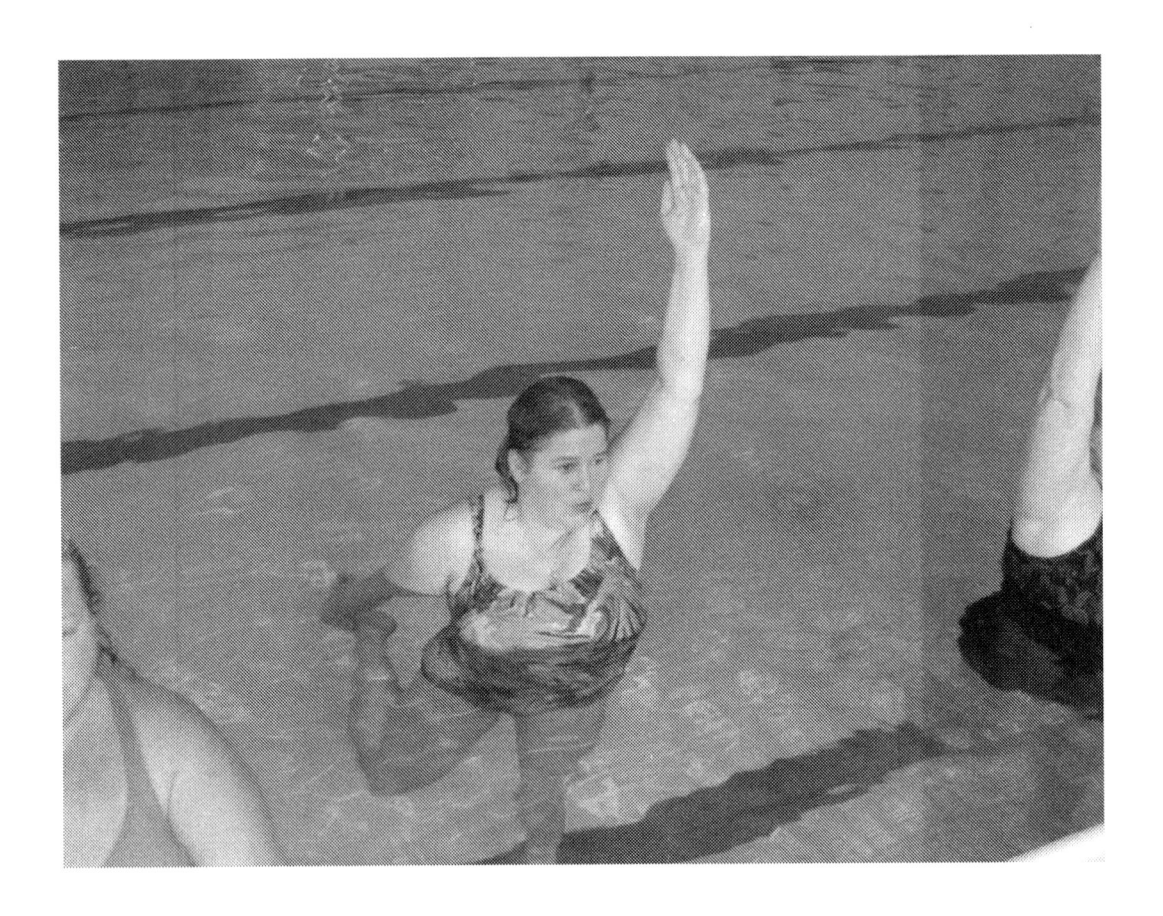

4- Arms Extended Overhead

KEY STUDENT INSTRUCTIONS

-Toes facing the pool wall
-Legs straight
-Extend arms overhead, palms facing each other
-Shoulders down

POOLSIDE TEACHER NOTES

-Arms inline with the ears if accessible
-Armpits deep and fingers together
-Broaden upper back
-Spreading shoulder blades

Work in Asana or Variations:

-Interlace fingers, palms upward and bend to the right on the exhale.
-Inhale come back to center
-Exhale bend to the left
-Inhale come back to center, etc.

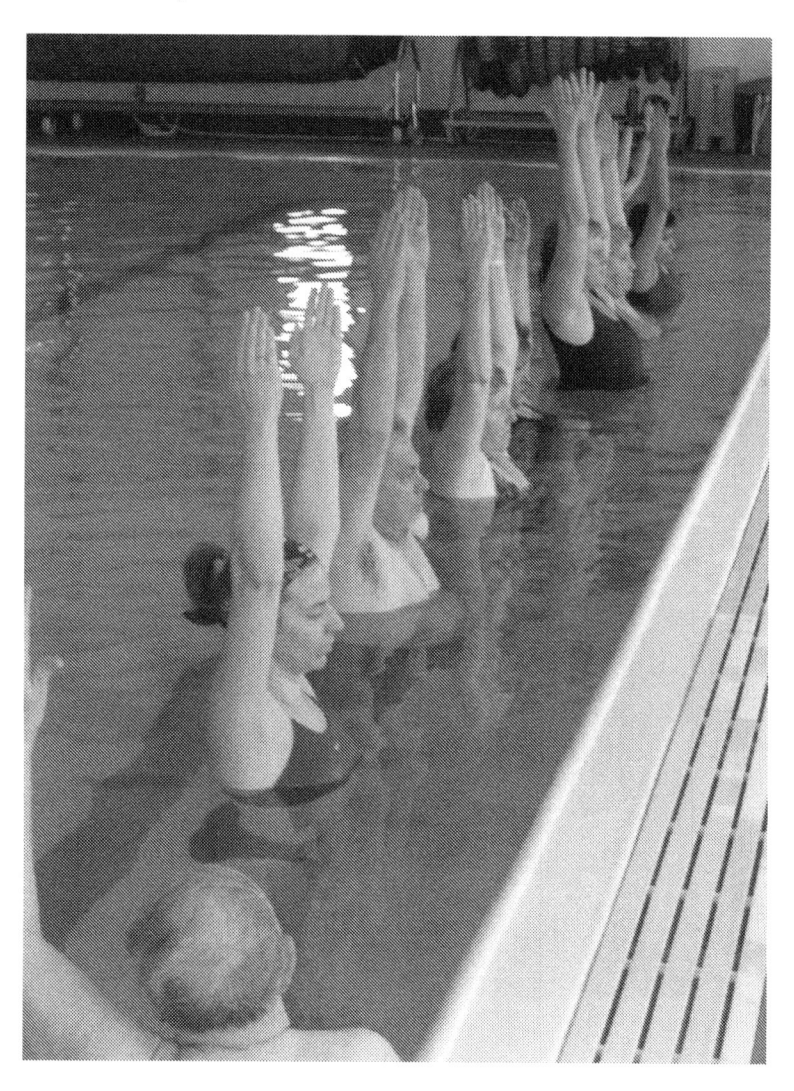

5- Fierce Pose

KEY STUDENT INSTRUCTIONS

-From Mountain Pose, raise the arms overhead, palms facing.
-Sink back into the back of an imaginary chair bending the knees.

POOLSIDE TEACHER NOTES

-Armpits deep
-Chin not jutting forwards, keep neck long.
-Knees same distance as hips.
-Draw shoulder blades open and down

Work in Asana or Variations:

-Instead of taking arms overhead, try resting the outer hands on the pool deck and draw in through the armpits, keeping shoulders down. Nice alternative if arms overhead not possible.
-From chair position, bring the right hand into sacrum and twist to right.
-Hold position and breathe into the right collarbone.
-Then release and try to the other side.

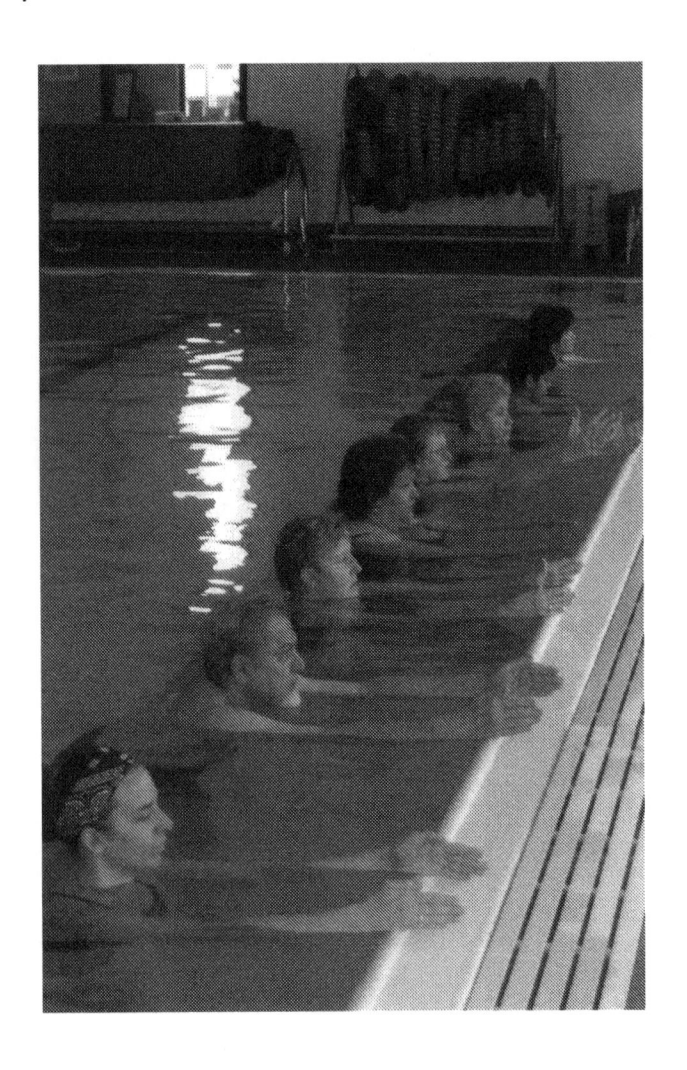

6-Warrior 1

KEY STUDENT INSTRUCTIONS

-Extend right toes up the pool wall with heel to the floor.
-Bend right knee 90 degrees
-Left leg extends back and up on toes.
-Extend 1 or both arms overhead. Palms facing
-Repeat to left side.

POOLSIDE TEACHER NOTES

-Top shoulders down
-Shin vertical

-Extend out through heel.
-Deep armpits. Sit bones moving down.

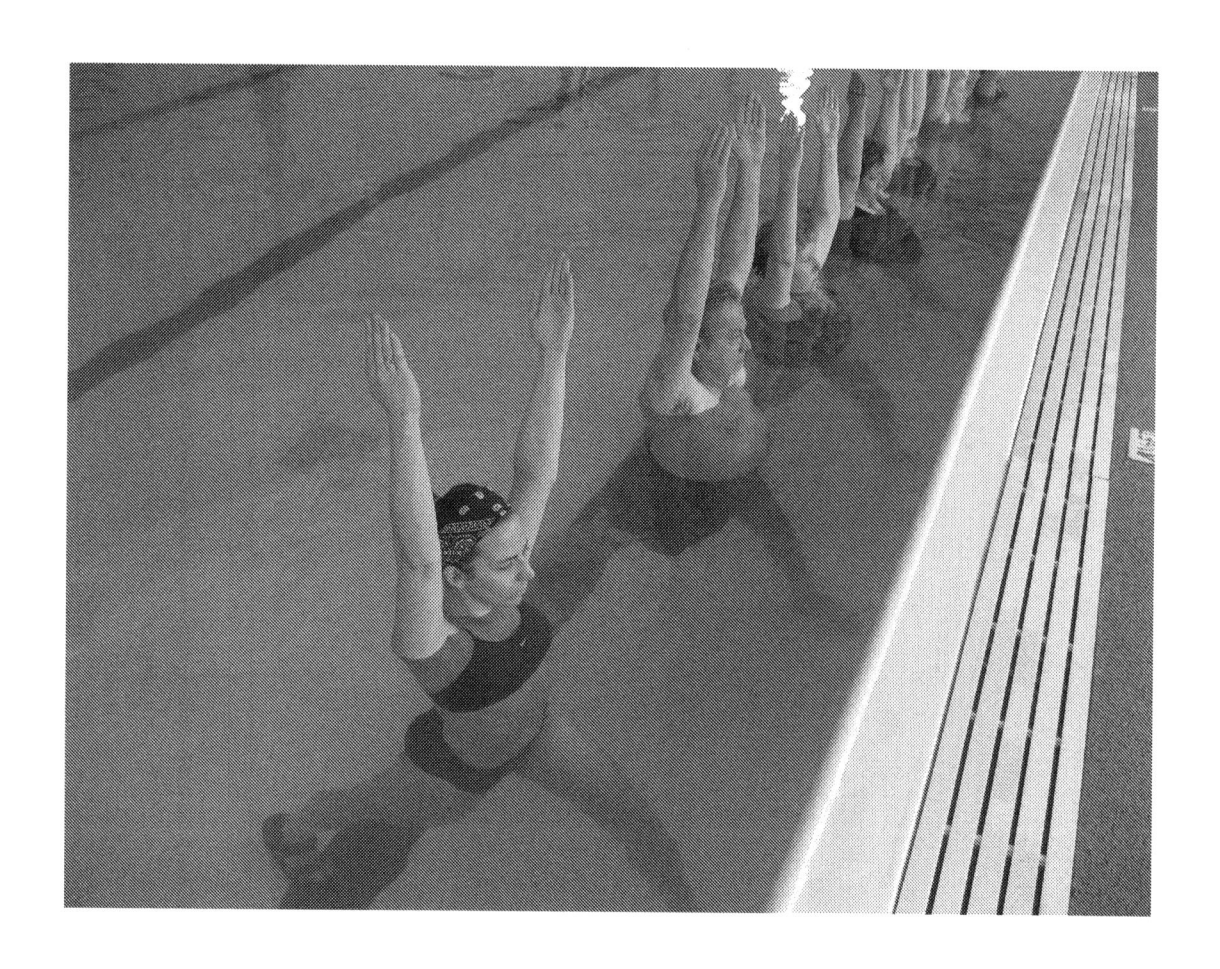

Work in Asana or Variations:

-From lunge put right hand to sacrum and twist from belly to right.
-Breathe into top right collarbone and draw shoulders down.
-Repeat to left

-From lunge with right foot to wall, turn left toes out to 10 on clock face as right toes are at 12.
-Sink down through back heel. Leg strong
-Draw left shoulder forward, squaring chest to pool wall.
-Keep sit bones down.
-Repeat to left

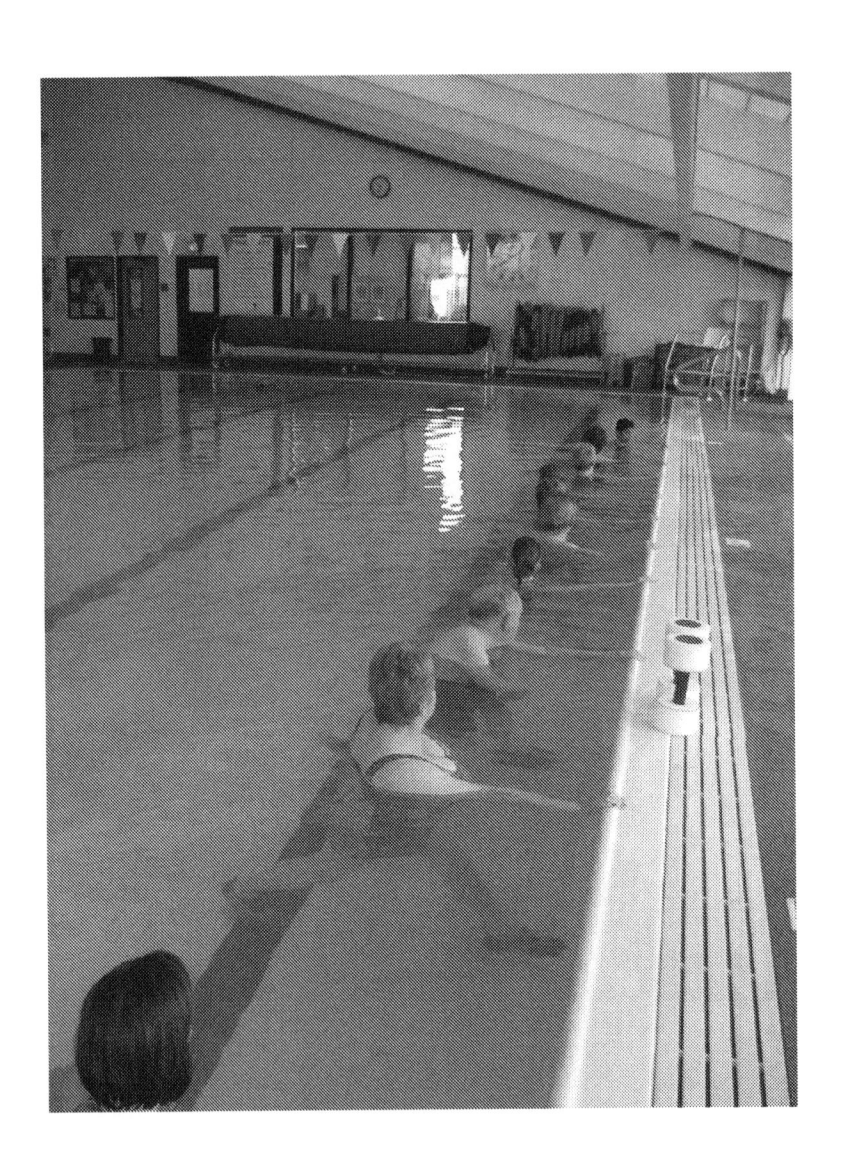

7- Walking Warrior

This is useful to get moving if the body temperature is a bit on the cool side. It challenges the breath and the body coordination in the water. It is much more difficult than it looks. Also, it is good to help with concentration and focus. It gives the teacher time to assess the class also.

KEY STUDENT INSTRUCTIONS

-Walking from one side of the pool to the other.
-Extend arms overhead. Can use float here if available.
-Exhale and step right foot forward, and lunge.
-Inhale and step left leg through.
-Repeat to the other side.

POOLSIDE TEACHER NOTES

-Arms straight if possible
-Tops shoulders down.
-Lift from waist.

Work in Asana or Variations:

-If you are too deep in the water, you may not be able to lunge very deeply. An alternative is to exhale and draw the knee up to the chest.
-Work on breathing patterning to fully exhale and fully inhale.
-Rest as needed

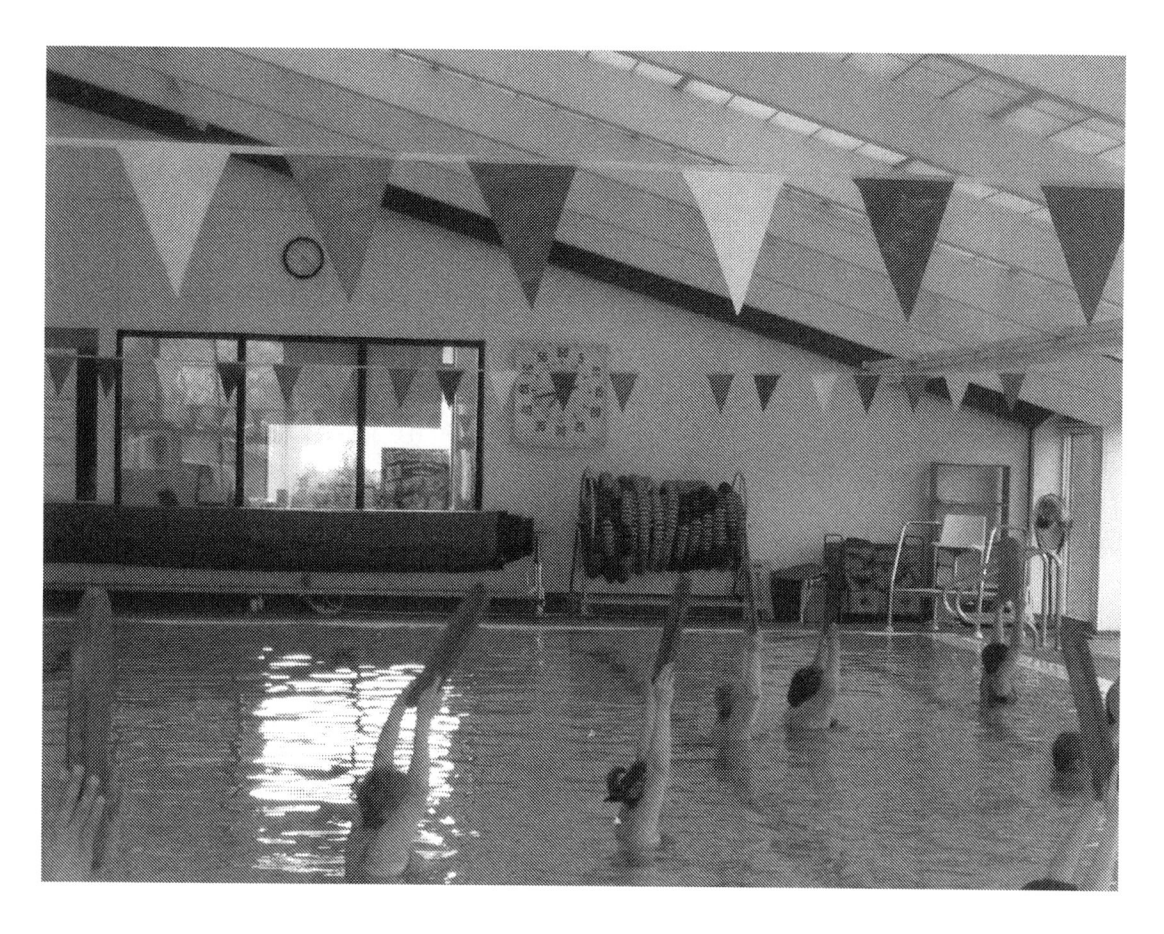

8 – Torso lengthening pose

KEY STUDENT INSTRUCTIONS

-Hold onto pool wall, hands shoulder width apart
-Push hips to other side of the pool, lengthening trunk.
-Legs straight if possible.

POOLSIDE TEACHER NOTES

-Hips over ankles. Groins deep.
-Armpits deep.
-Shoulders down.

Work in Asana or Variations:

-Right leg steps forward. Toes up wall.
-Pull Right hip back and lengthen Right side
-Both legs straight if possible or front leg bent.
-R hand on sacrum, push down through back heel and twist to Right from belly.
-Thorasic moves in. Length to front.
-Check length both sides trunk.

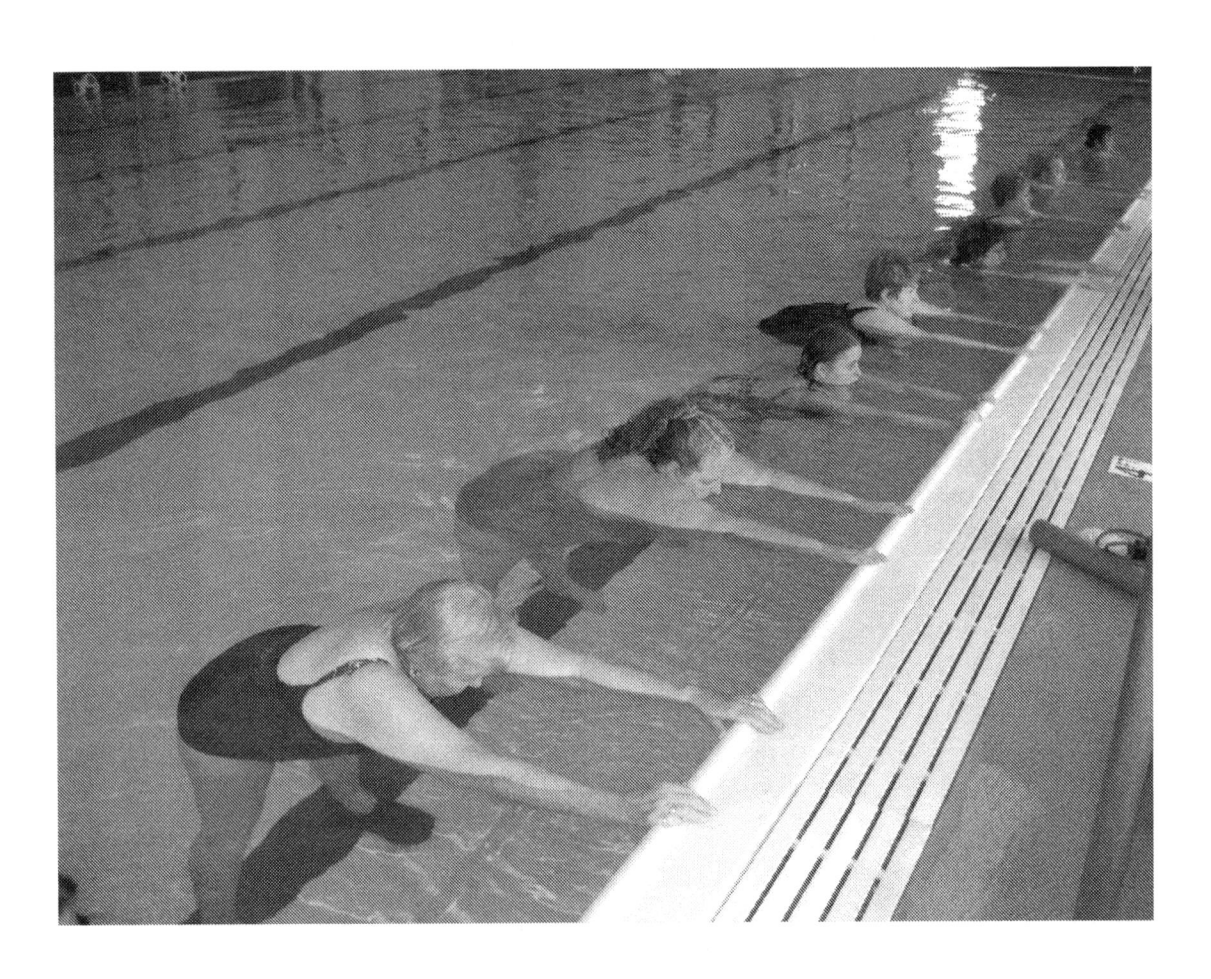

9- Stabilize shoulders

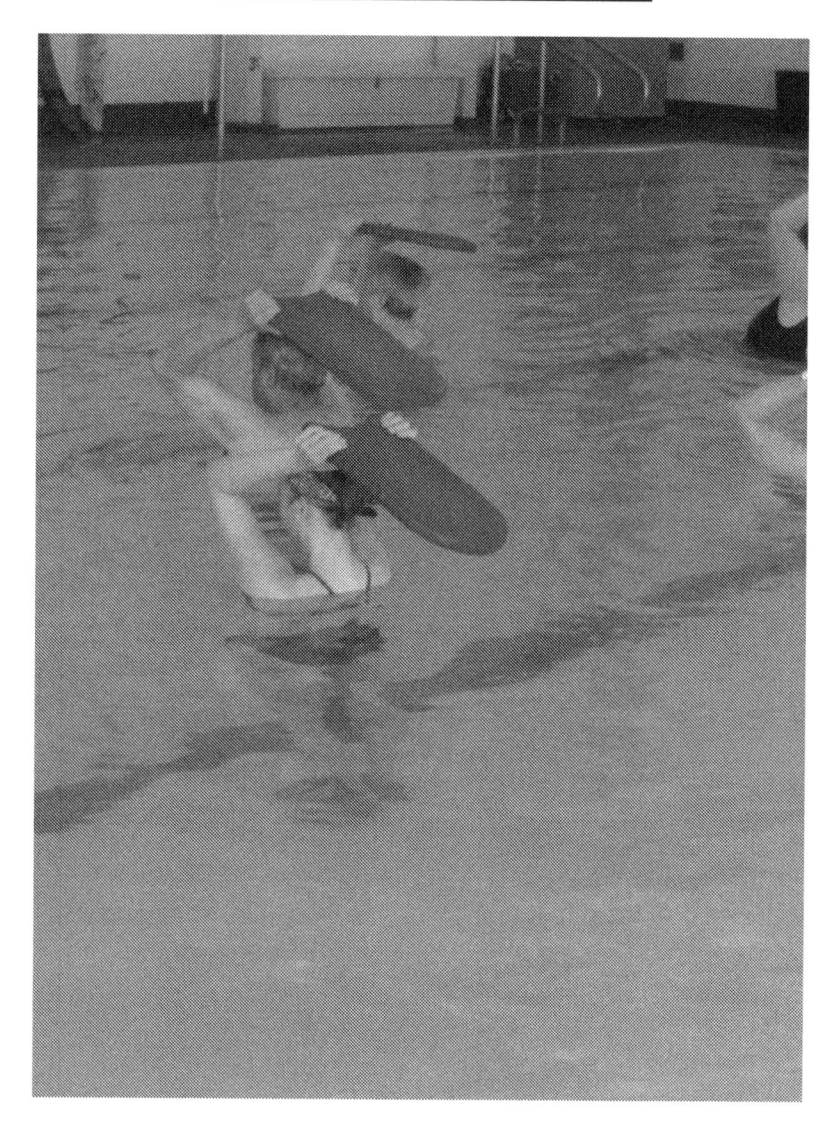

KEY STUDENT INSTRUCTIONS

-Hold float overhead between palms of hands and bend elbows.
-Keep elbows facing fwd and shoulders down.

Work in Asana or Variations:

-Try walking to the other side holding the float overhead.
-Keep shoulders stable and breath nice and even.
-Rest when needed

POOLSIDE TEACHER NOTES

-Elbows in, armpits deep. Shoulders down
-Length and breath to back body.
-Chin in.
-Spine long. Legs strong.

9A-More Shoulder Work

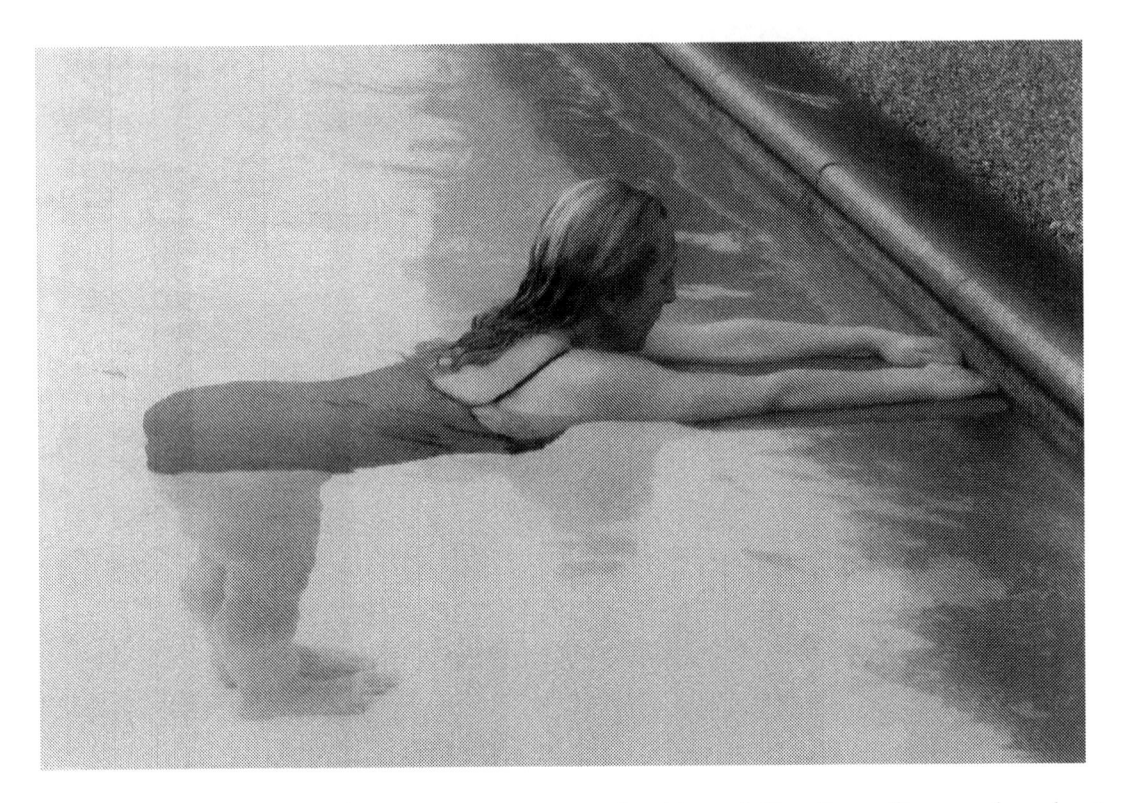

Try using the resistance in the water to gain greater shoulder stability. Start of in torso lengthening pose. Keep shoulders down and elbows in and move hips forwards. Bringing float to the ribs on the inhale. Exhale, and push hips back to original position. "Much harder than it looks!"

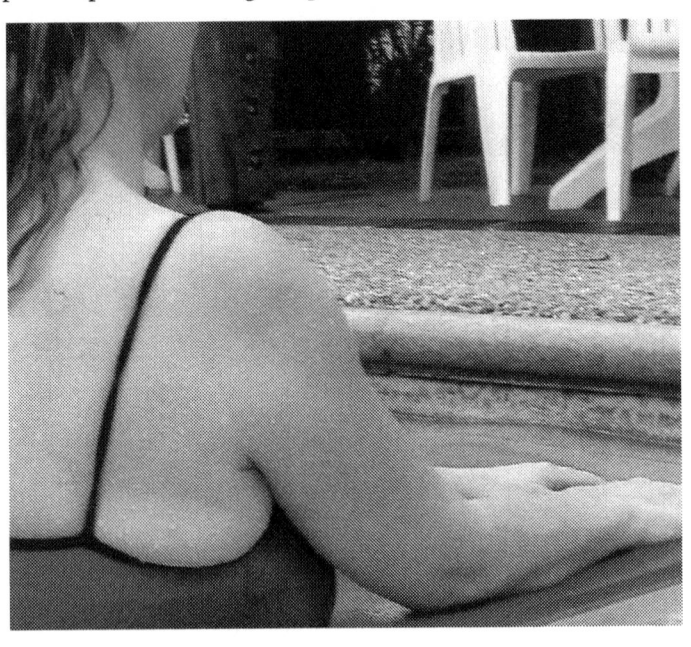

It works much like dolphin dips do on land, creating strength and stability.

10- Warrior 2 & Half Moon

Taking the toes up the pool wall motivates more work in the legs and feet that can be lacking in the pool.

It is also good for flat feet.

KEY STUDENT INSTRUCTIONS

-Face pool wall. Feet hip distance.
-Right toes up wall and Right hand to wall.
-Extend Left leg back, turn toes out and get heel to floor.
-Reach across pool with Left arm. Fingers together.
-Release the sit bones down.
-Repeat to other side.

POOLSIDE TEACHER NOTES

-Pigeon toed on back leg. So heel out.
-Shoulders down arms same height
-Length to front and back torso.
-Check bent knee above ankle.

Work in Asana or Variations:

-From Warrior 2, Right leg forward, lift Left leg and extend Left heel to other side of pool.
-Raise Left arm to ceiling.
-Straighten Right leg.
-Repeat to other side.
-Both legs straight and in line with back body.
-Floating ribs in.

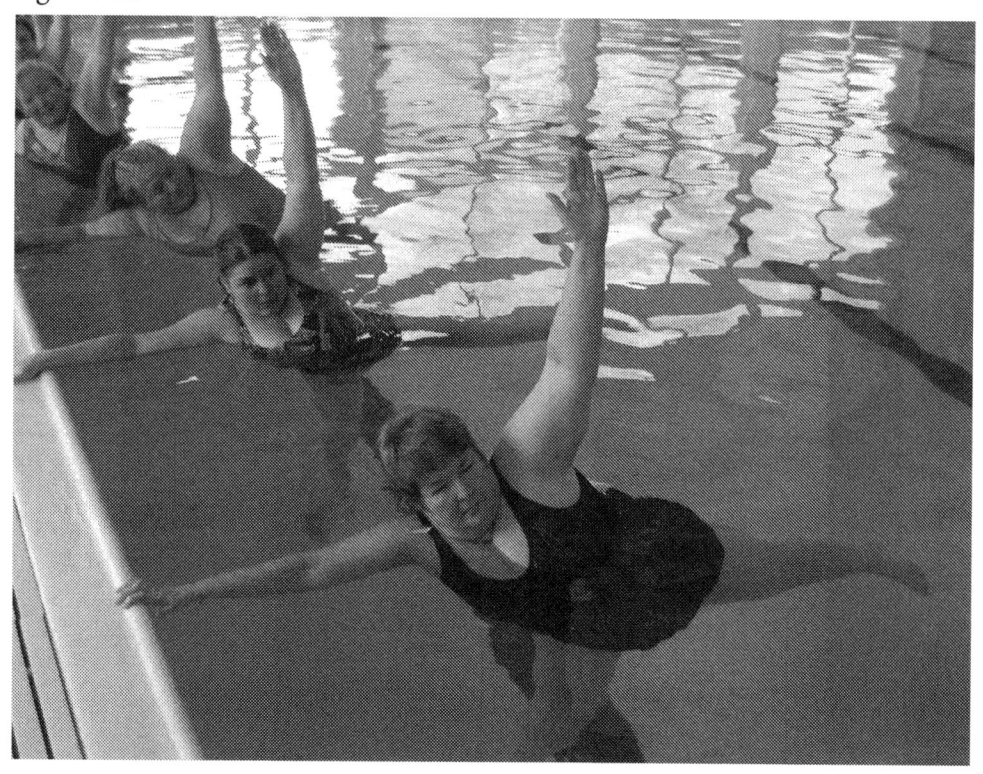

Half Moon Pose. This confident pose can be held by a wider audience than on land.

Warrior 2 pose

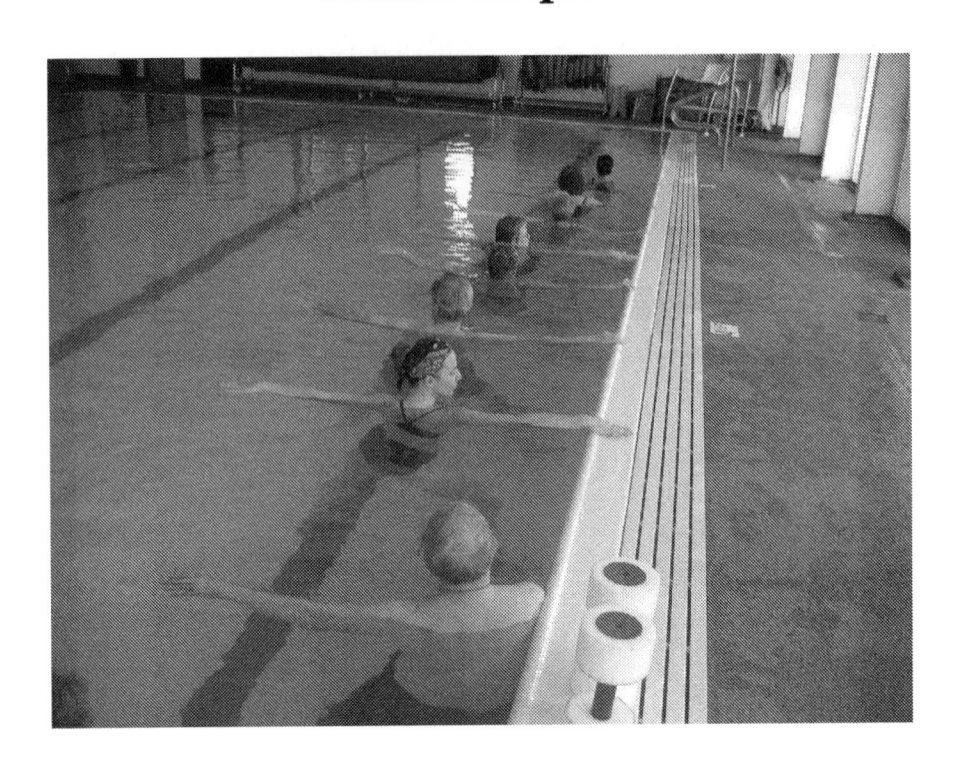

Half Moon

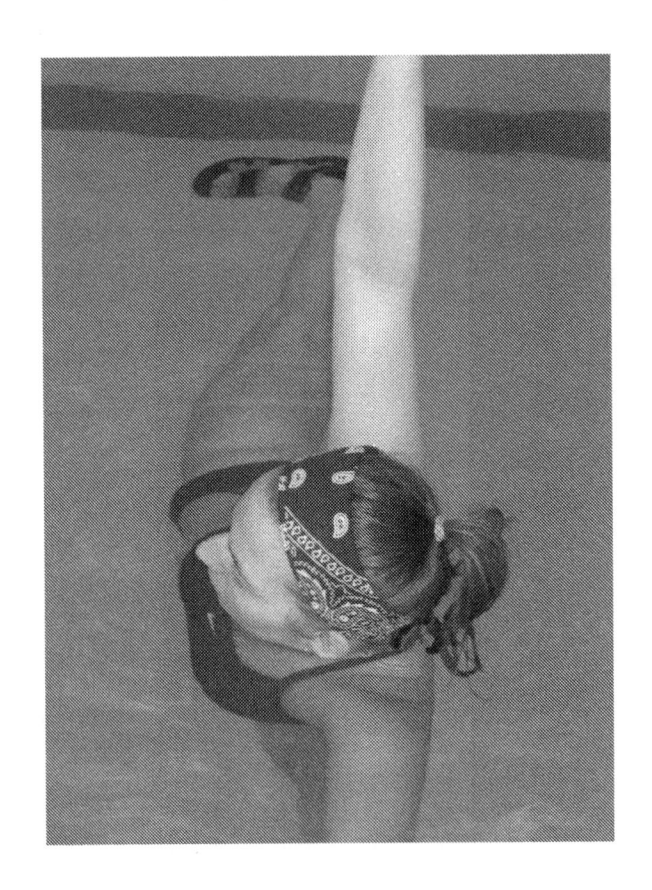

11- Lateral Angle Pose & Triangle Pose

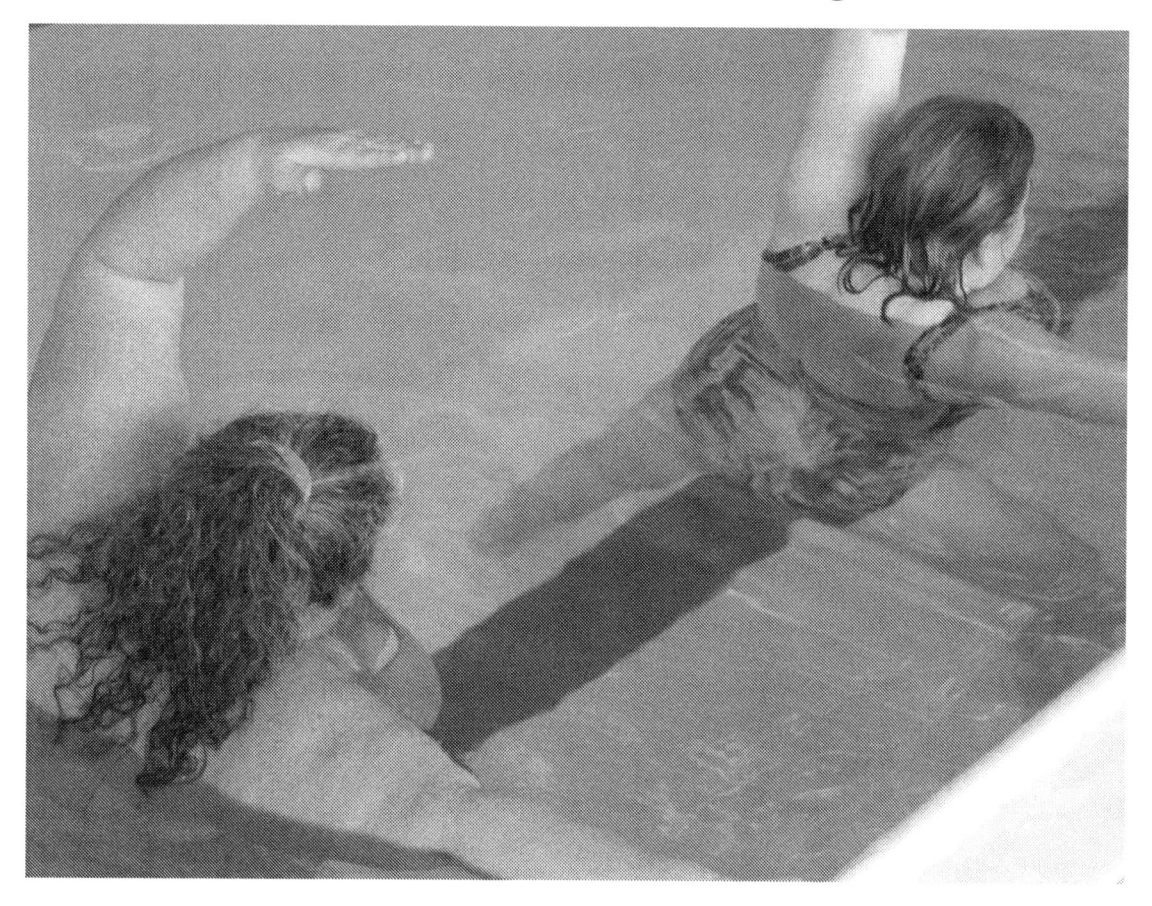

KEY STUDENT INSTRUCTIONS

-Face pool wall. Feet hip distance.
-Step Right foot forward. Toes up wall
-Right hand to wall.
-Bend Right knee to Right angles. Shin vertical.
-Extend Left leg back and turn toes out. Heel in.
-Extend Left arm overhead like a rainbow.
-Palm down.
-Repeat to Left side.

POOLSIDE TEACHER NOTES

-Rotate trunk to Left.
-Tail bone untucked.
-Sit bones down
-Deep armpit.

Work in Asana or Variations:

Adding movement in the asana:
-Inhaling and extending left arm out with the palm face up.
-Exhaling and taking arm close to ear.
-Full inhalation and full exhalation.
-Repeat several times, then switch sides.

Triangle Pose and Half Moon Pose Options:
-Moving to triangle from here by straightening Right leg, and extending Left arm to ceiling.
  -Moving to Half Moon, but may need to step away from the wall to keep Right arm straight.

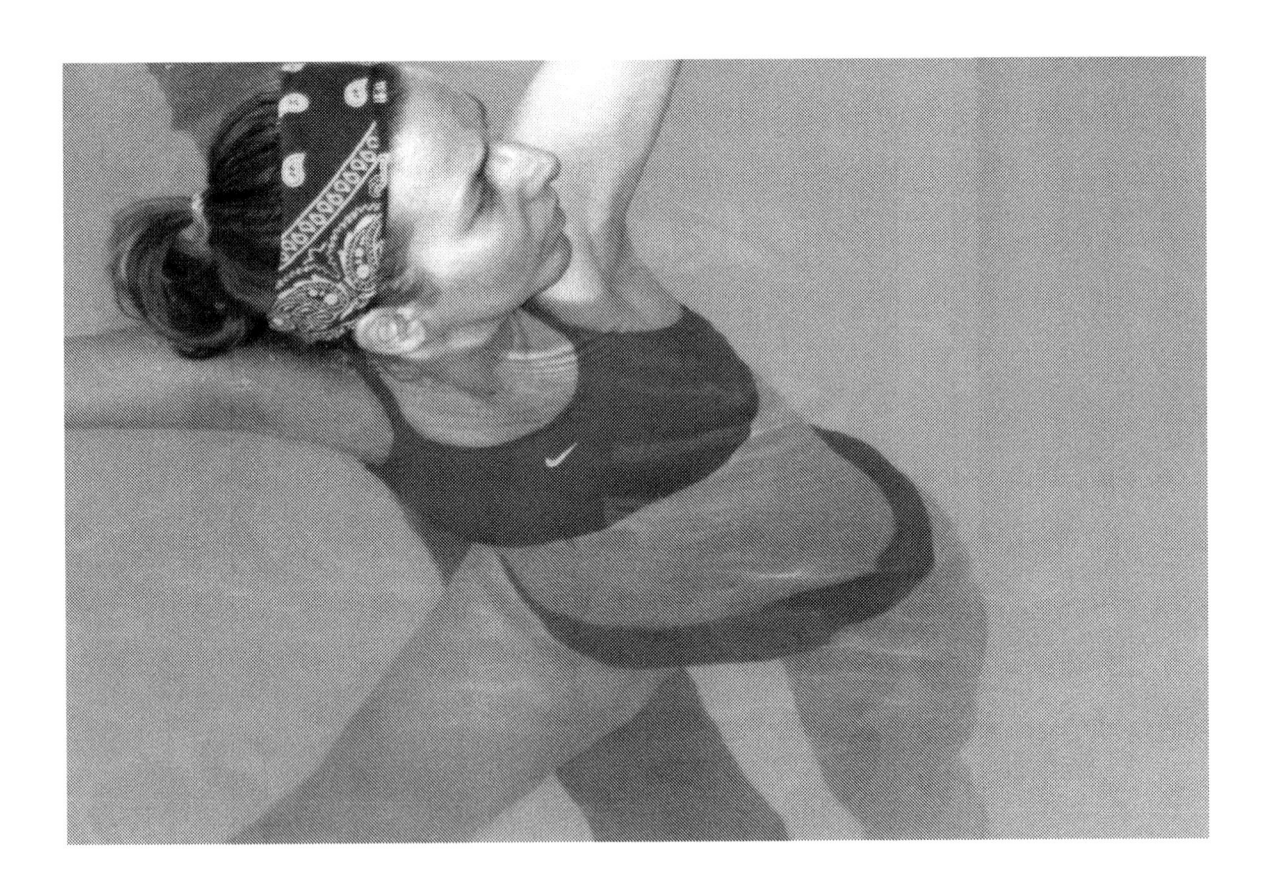

12- Straight Leg & Reverse Twist

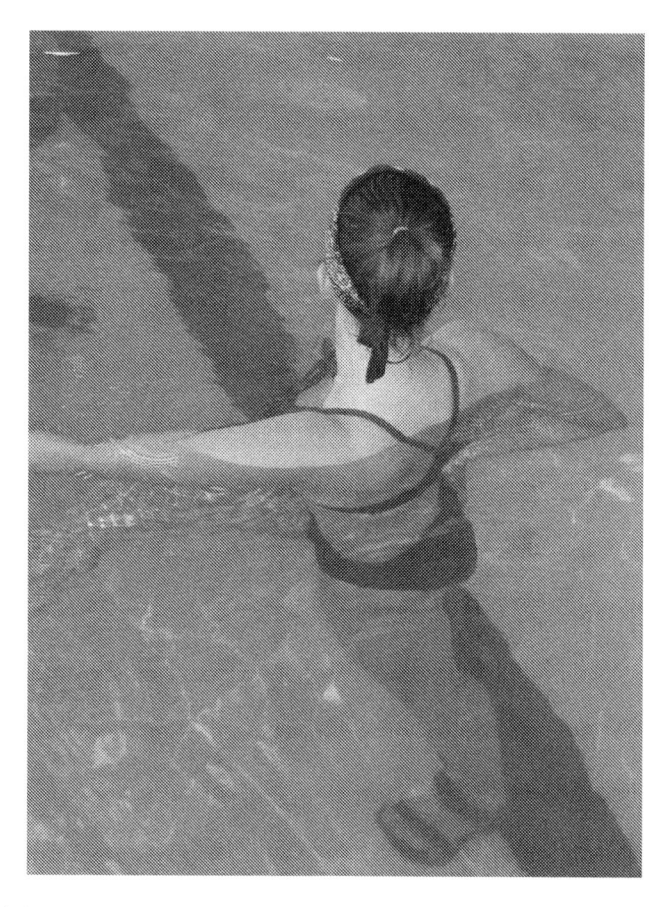

KEY STUDENT INSTRUCTIONS

-Step away from pool wall enough to allow sole of Right foot to push into pool wall.
-Both legs straight, or at least supporting leg straight. -Extend both arms overhead. Palms facing.
-Lengthen the spine with the breath.
-Repeat to Left leg.

POOLSIDE TEACHER NOTES

-Hips same height.
-Toes and knee facing upwards.
-Shoulders down.
-Deep armpits.

Work in Asana or Variations:

-Bend Right knee and bring Right hand to sacrum.
-Rotate from belly to Right, keeping shoulders down.
-Soften inner body.
-If hamstrings allow hold twist and straighten Right leg.
-Keep supporting leg strong.
-Chin parallel to water.
-Check breath integrity.

13- Horse Stance

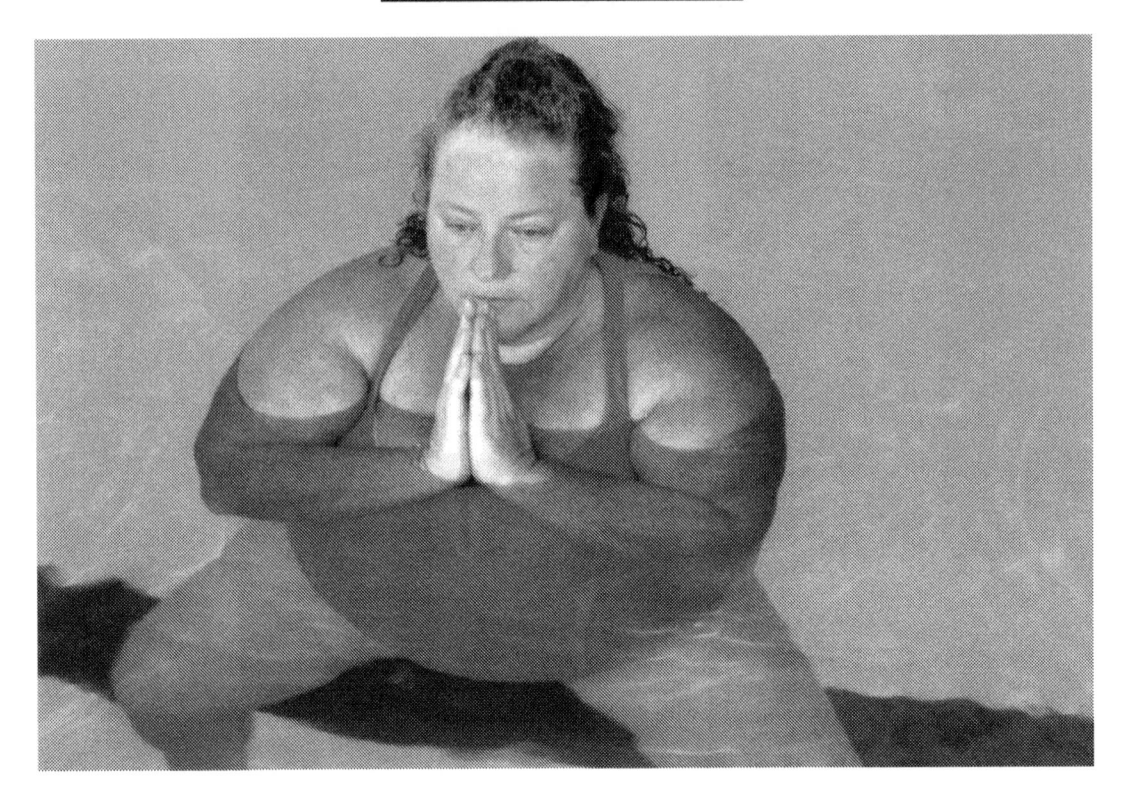

Horse stance is just a nice gentle way to open up the hips.

KEY STUDENT INSTRUCTIONS

-Face wall and step feet wider than hips.
-Turn toes out 45 degrees or wider.
-Keeping spine vertical and untuck sitbones
-Bend knees into a squat as you exhale.
-Hands onto pool or across the heart in prayer position.

Work in Asana or Variations:

Work with the breath:
-Exhale and squat
-Inhale and stand up

-Can have back to wall also.

POOLSIDE TEACHER NOTES

-Open chest
-Sit bones down. Don't stick butt out.
-Shoulders back and down.

14- Rainbow Shoulder Rotations

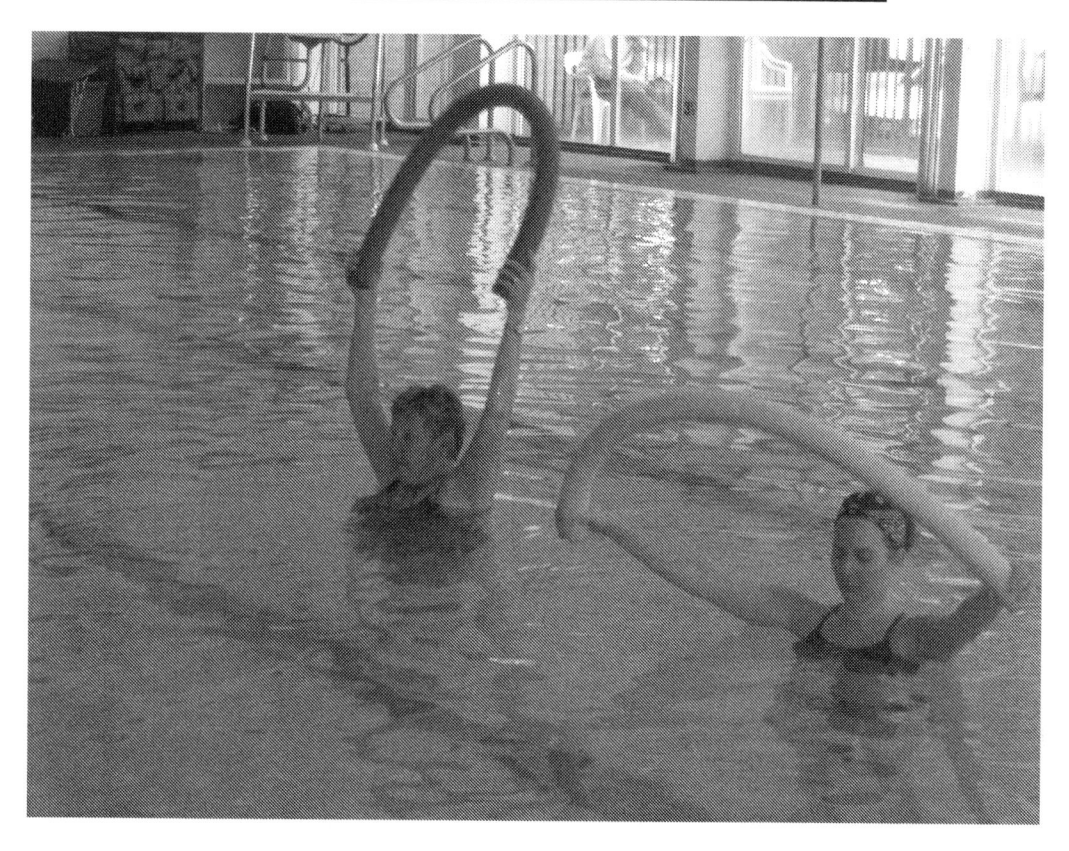

14. Foam noodles can be a useful prop for the aqua yoga students.

KEY STUDENT INSTRUCTIONS

-Hold noodle in both hands wider than shoulders.
-Inhale, and extend arms overhead as far as you can.
-Exhale, and bring arms back down in front.

POOLSIDE TEACHER NOTES

-Rotate shoulders if possible.
-Keep hands wide to get maximum shoulder rotation.

Work in Asana or Variations:

-Try to extend the length of inhale and exhale.
-If body temperature is on the cool side, try walking across pool at the same time. Need to focus more.

15- Plank Pose & Side Plank Pose

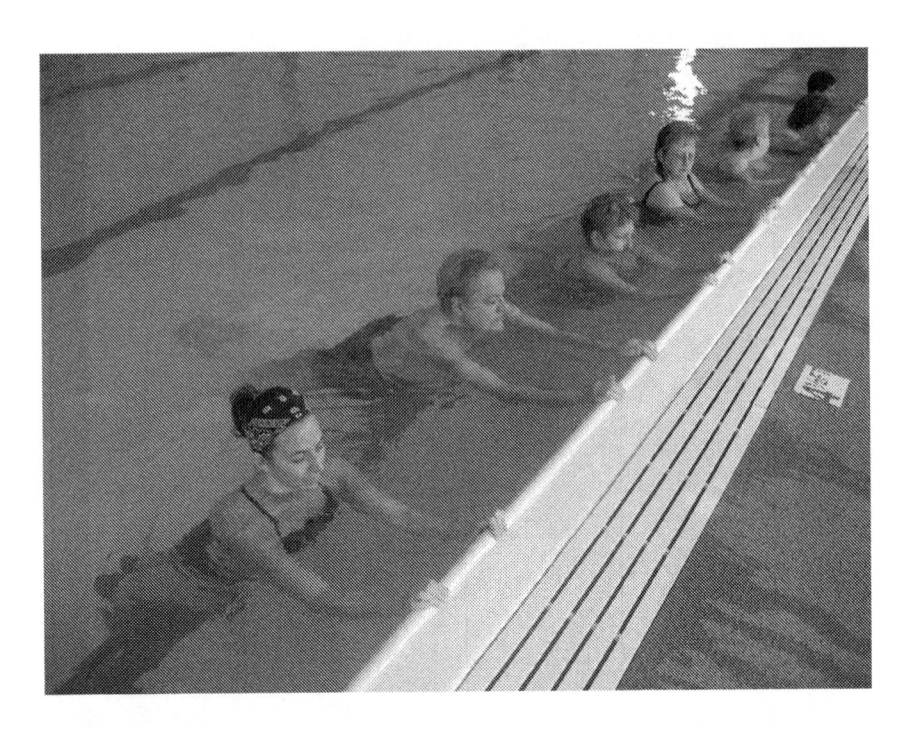

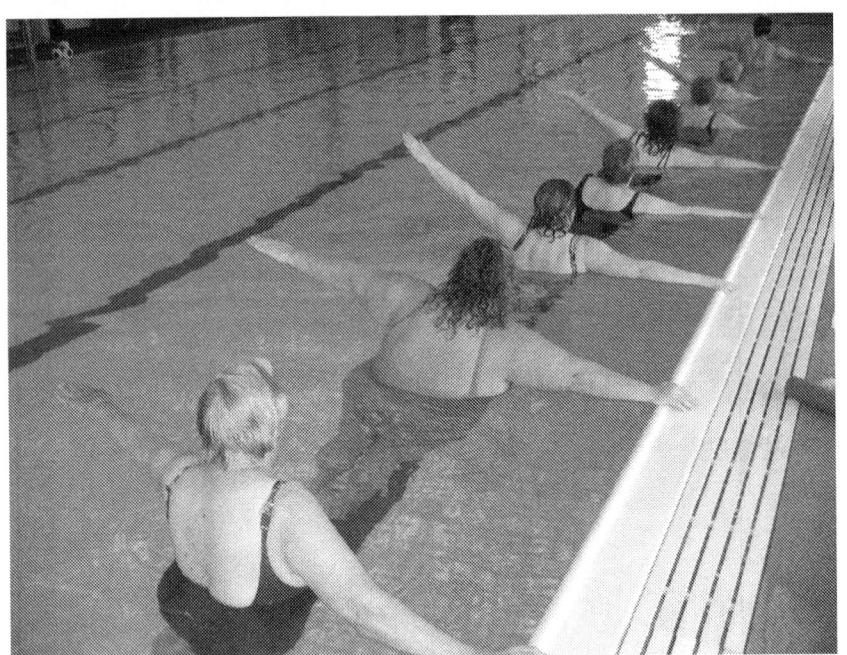

KEY STUDENT INSTRUCTIONS

Stand away from pool wall holding on to side. Come up on to toes and push out through heels. Back of body in a straight line Lift heart.
For side Plank open up to one side and reach across the pool with arm.

POOLSIDE TEACHER NOTES

. Neck long and arms, wrists shoulder width,
. Shoulders down and armpits deep. Step back further if butt sticks out.
Try to keep shoulders same height.

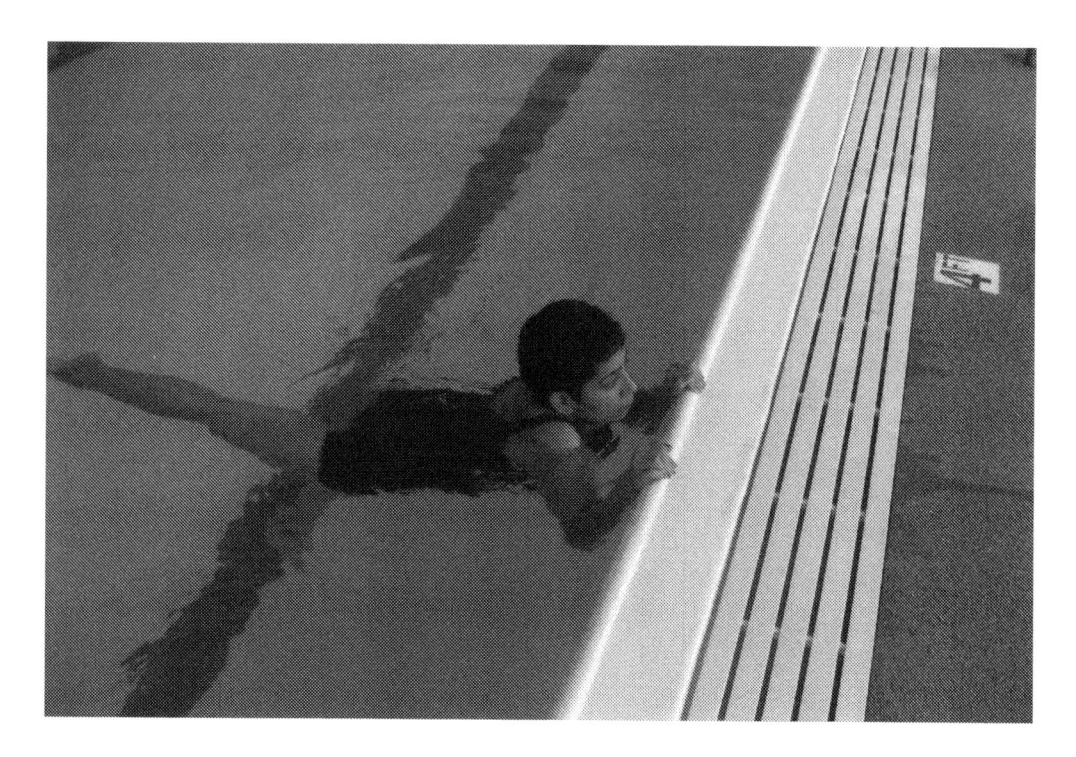

Plank Variation taking elbows to pool wall during exhale, 1 leg raised.

Work in Asana or Variations:
-Lift Right leg behind and keep it straight.
-Repeat the other side.

Working on breath count:
-Inhale raise the leg.
-Exhale lower the leg.
-Switch legs

-Exhale: Keep elbows in, and bring forearms to pool wall.
-Inhale: Straighten the arms.
-Can also raise one leg, or both legs through the sequence.
-Make sure shoulders are stable.
-Keep heart lifted and shoulders down.

-*In the picture* : **Plank Variation**:
Taking the elbows to pool wall during exhale. One leg lifted is also another variation. Inhale straightening the arms and bring the foot back on the floor.

16 – Eagle Pose

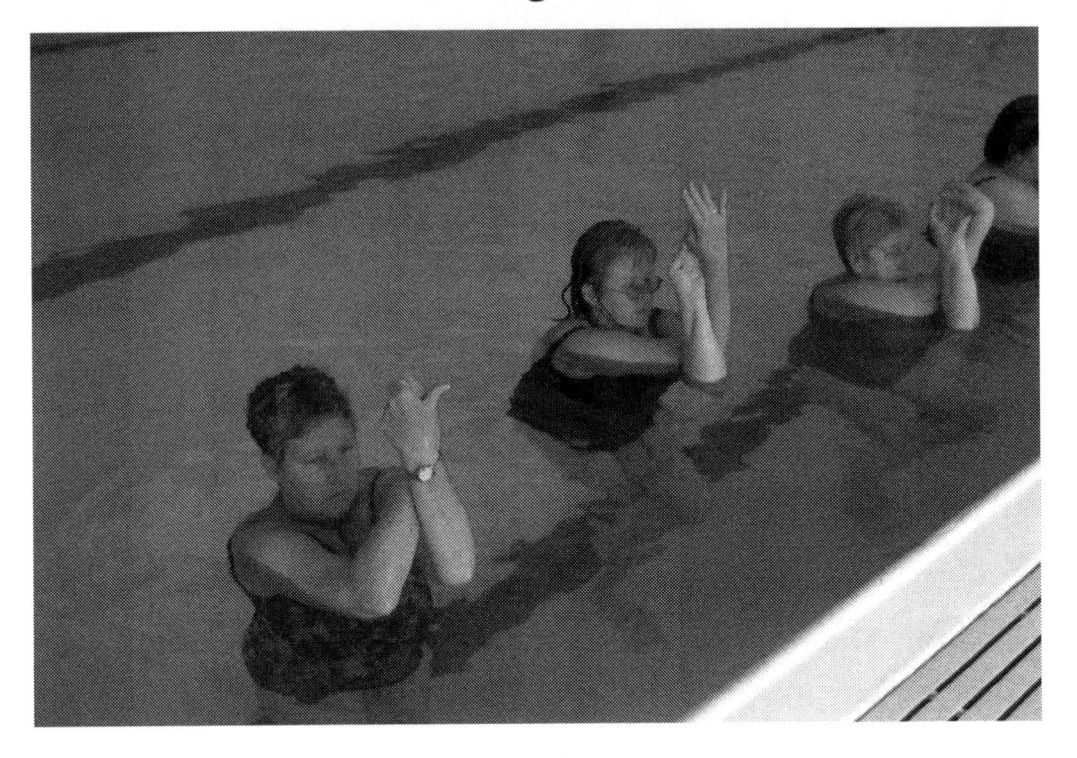

Eagle Pose

KEY STUDENT INSTRUCTIONS

-Arms extend in front.
-Cross Right arm over Left., Shoulders down.
-Bend elbows, and try to bring hands together.
-Cross Left leg over Right, and sit back into imaginary chair.
-Repeat to other side.

Work in Asana or Variations:

-If not happy with arm position try bringing palms together in prayer position.
-Aiming at bringing elbows together.

POOLSIDE TEACHER NOTES

-Shoulders down.
-Breathe into back body.

17- Simple Backbend

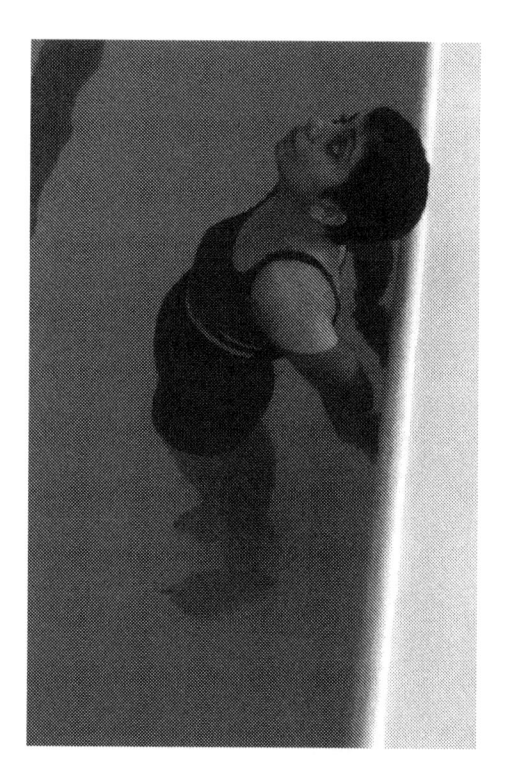

Simple Back Bend Variation

KEY STUDENT INSTRUCTIONS

-Face pool wall in Mountain pose.
-Hands to pool side.
-Inhale raise Right arm, palm faces Left
-Push hips forward and hold for a few breaths.
-Repeat to other side.

Work in Asana or Variations:
-Inhale: Raise arm
-Exhale: Arms down.
-Repeat to other side.

-Back to pool wall.
-Take shoulders back and bring palms to pool wall.
-Push hips forward and look up.
-Hold for a few breaths.
-Try chin to chest for variation. Lengthen back of neck.
-Lift the heart. Shoulders down.
-Possible assist from teacher to bring shoulders in, towards one another.

POOLSIDE TEACHER NOTES

-Legs very firm.
-Heels apart. No duck feet.
-Look up if comfortable.
-Lengthen front and back spine.

18- Tree Balance

Balance poses can become much more accessible in the water than on land, but not if the water is agitated. Student can practice with back to the wall, facing the wall, or "bent branch" leg gently touching pool wall.

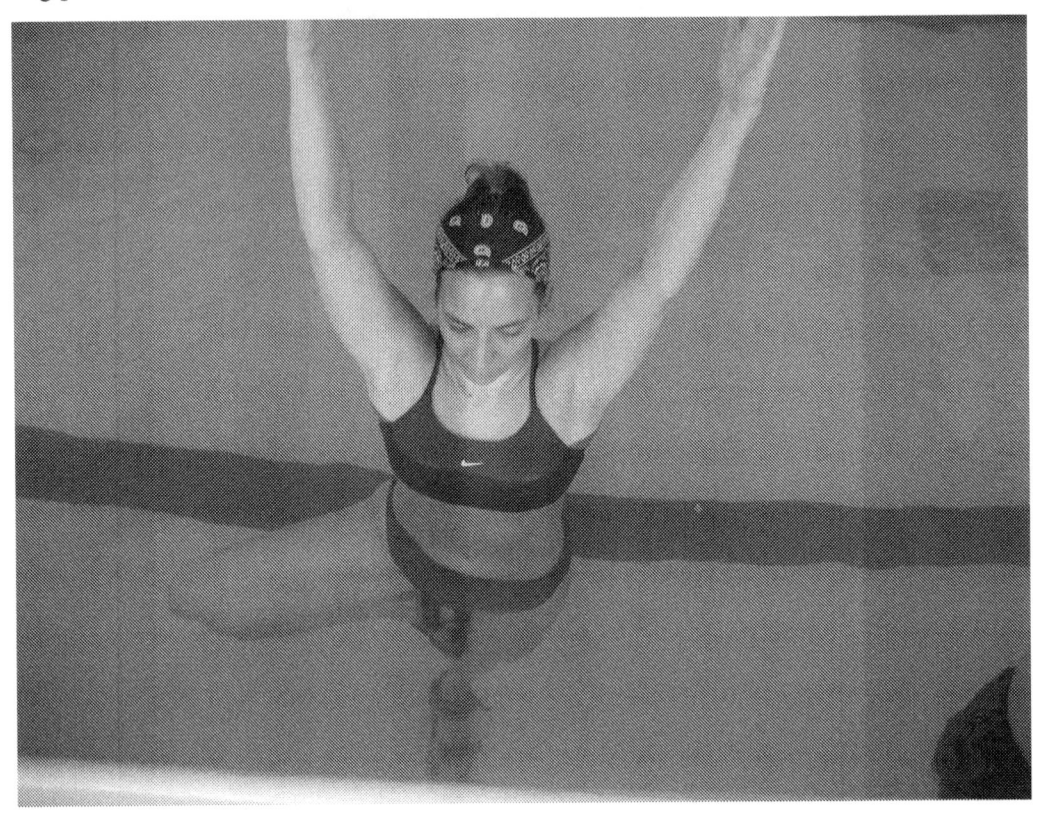

18. Tree Balance

KEY STUDENT INSTRUCTIONS

-Bring sole of Right foot to inner Left leg.
-Opening Right hip joint.
-Take one, or both arms overhead. Palms facing each other.
-Hold for a few breaths.
Repeat to other side.

POOLSIDE TEACHER NOTES

-Keep hips at same level.
 -Keep supporting leg strong.
 -Lengthen torso.

Work in Asana or Variations:

 -Can have hands together in prayer position.
 -Inhale taking arms up.
 -Exhale bringing arms down.
 -Try to bring hands together behind the back in prayer position.
 -Try bringing outer Right foot to front Left thigh, and sit back as if in a chair to open hip further.

19- Cobra Pose

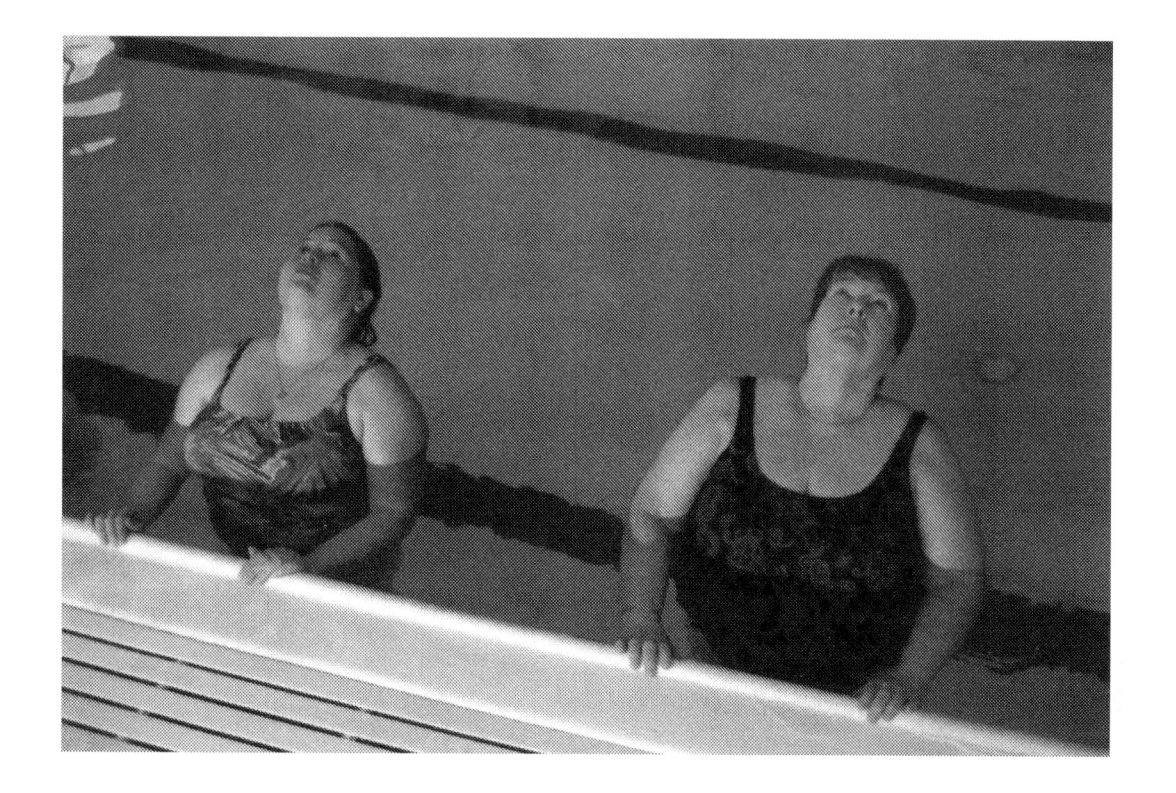

Cobra Pose

KEY STUDENT INSTRUCTIONS

-Facing wall, hold on wrists shoulder distance apart.
-Keep elbows in, and legs strong.
-Lead chest and hips forward, and look up.

Work in Asana or Variations:
-Try standing on toes, and straighten arms in back bend.
-Step feet out wide.
-Turn head to left then to right.
-Keep arms in, and shoulders down.

POOLSIDE TEACHER NOTES

-Some may step back further if o.k.

20- Tummy Toners

These exercises can be done with or without a foam noodle.

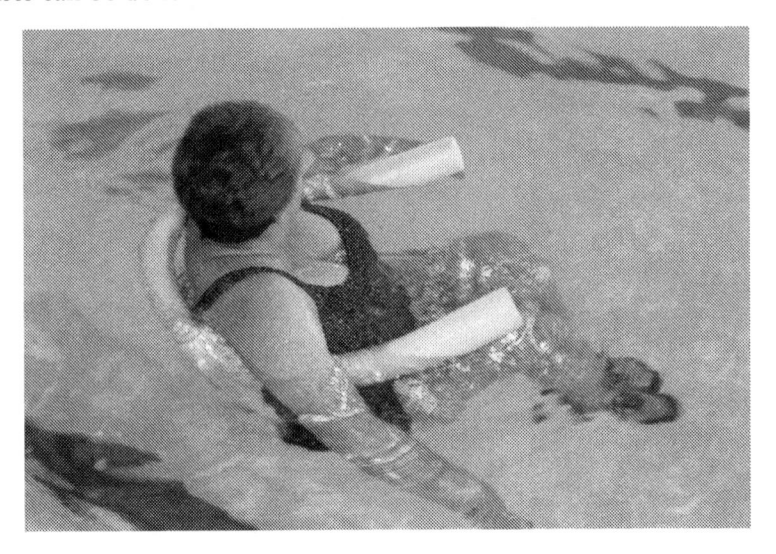

exhale pull knees into chest

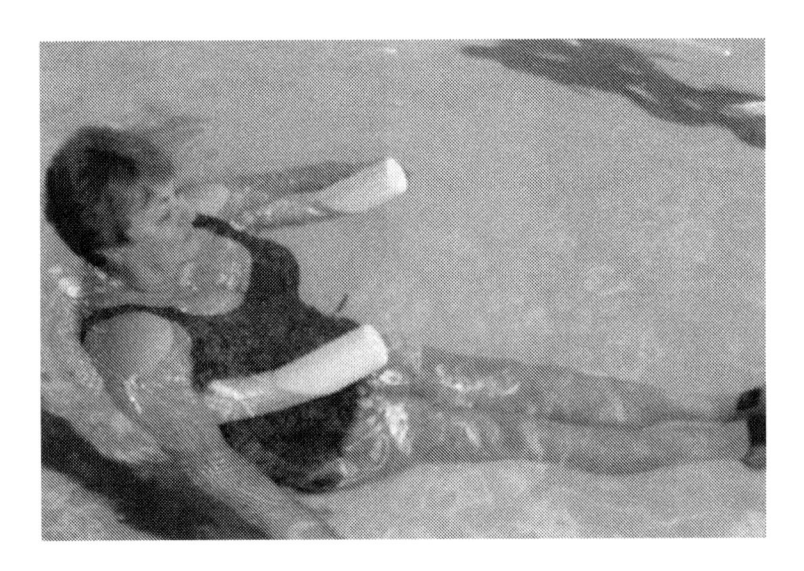

Inhale, extend legs out

KEY STUDENT INSTRUCTIONS

-Move away from pool wall.
-Place noodle under armpits.
-Exhale and draw knees to chest.
-Inhale and straighten legs in front.

Work in Asana or Variations:
-Can alternate legs in a cycling motion.

POOLSIDE TEACHER NOTES

-Shoulders down.
-Make sure breath awareness.

21- Groin Stretch & Hip Opener

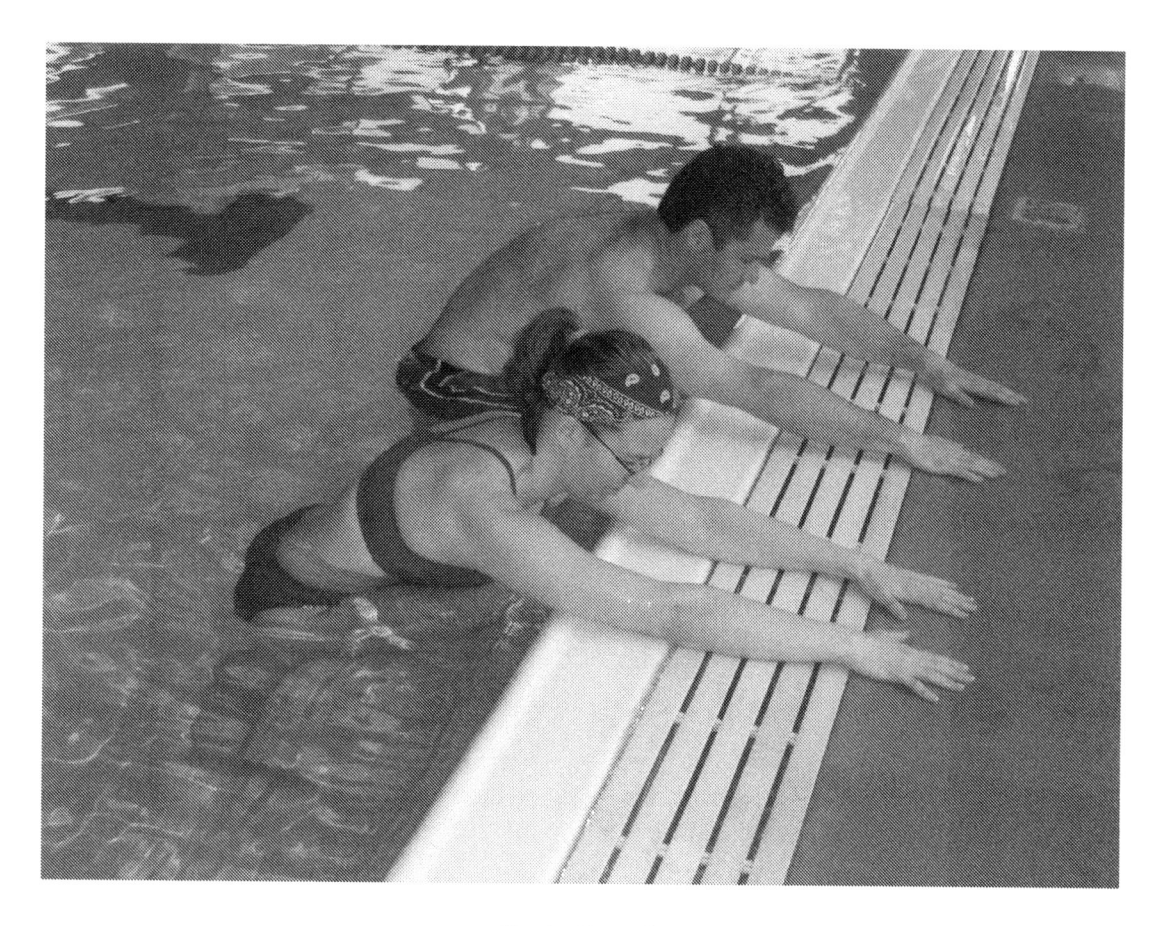

Groin Stretch

KEY STUDENT INSTRUCTIONS

-Face pool wall and bring shin to midline chest.
-Lengthen Left side. Keep shoulders down.
-Breathe well.
-Lengthen belly.
-Repeat to other side.

POOLSIDE TEACHER NOTES

-Extend the arms to deck to secure position.
-Neck and extension of the spine.

21- Groin Stretch & Hip Opener

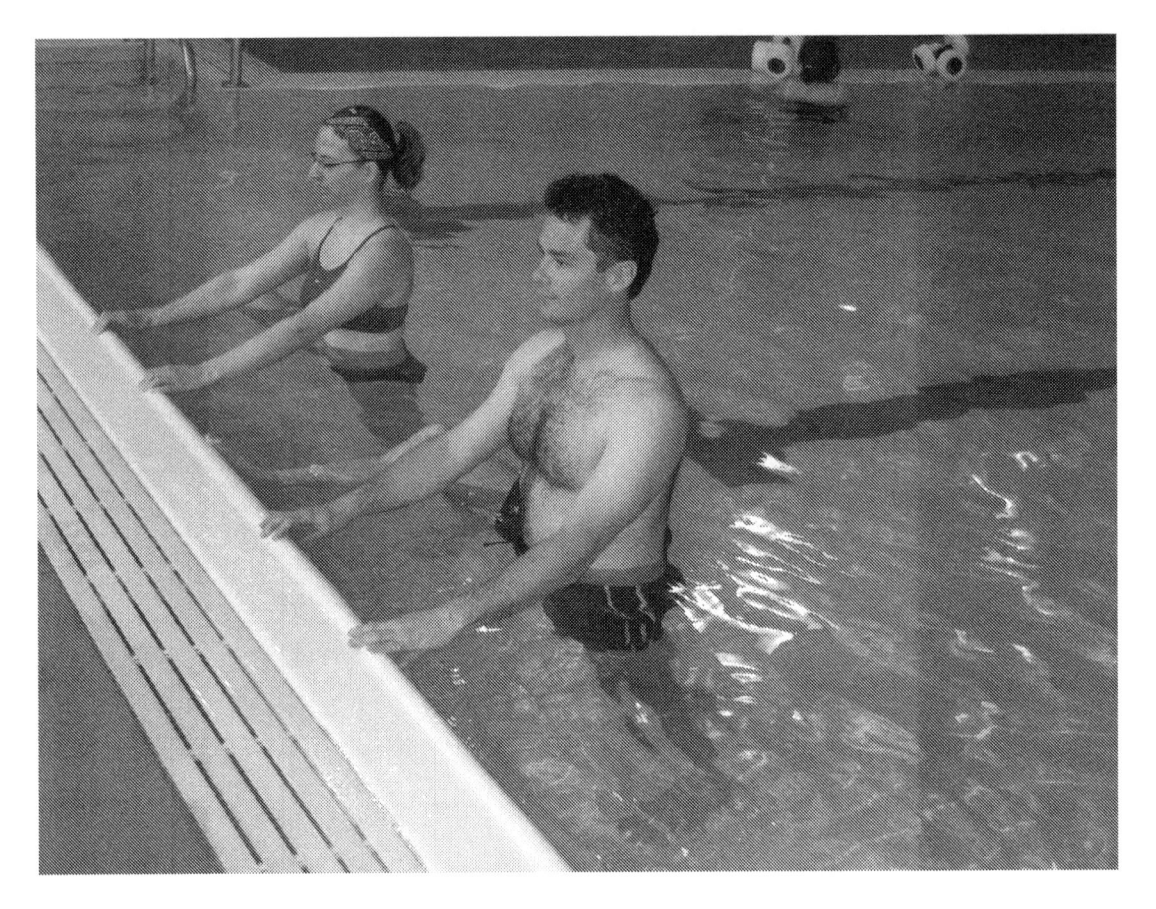

Hip Opener

Work in Asana or Variations:

-Place sole of Right foot to pool wall wider than hip.
-Bend Right knee but work Left leg straight.
-Lift heart and lengthen spine.
-Repeat to other side.
-Shoulders down and neck long.
-Hands, shoulder distance apart.

22- Noble Seal Pose

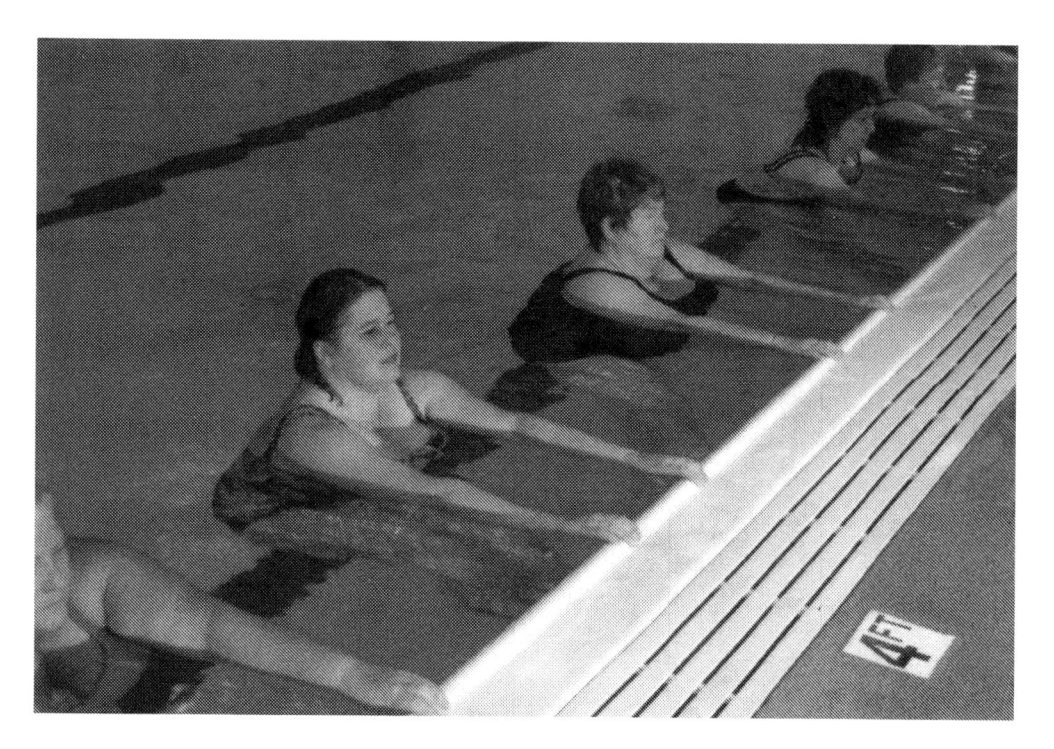

Noble Seal Pose

KEY STUDENT INSTRUCTIONS

-Hold on to pool wall. Hands shoulder width.
-Bring soles of feet to wall; hip distance or wider.
-Stay here and focus on breath with intensity.

POOLSIDE TEACHER NOTES

-Lift heart, shoulders down.
-Bring breath into sides of body.
-Try not to round lower back.
-Lengthen torso.

Work in Asana or Variations:

-Can play with the distance of the legs on wall.
-Keep integrity of breath and inner body length.
-Try bring outer Right foot into Left groin while keeping integrity of the breath, and inner body length.
-Repeat to other side.

23. Resting Pose or Corpse Pose

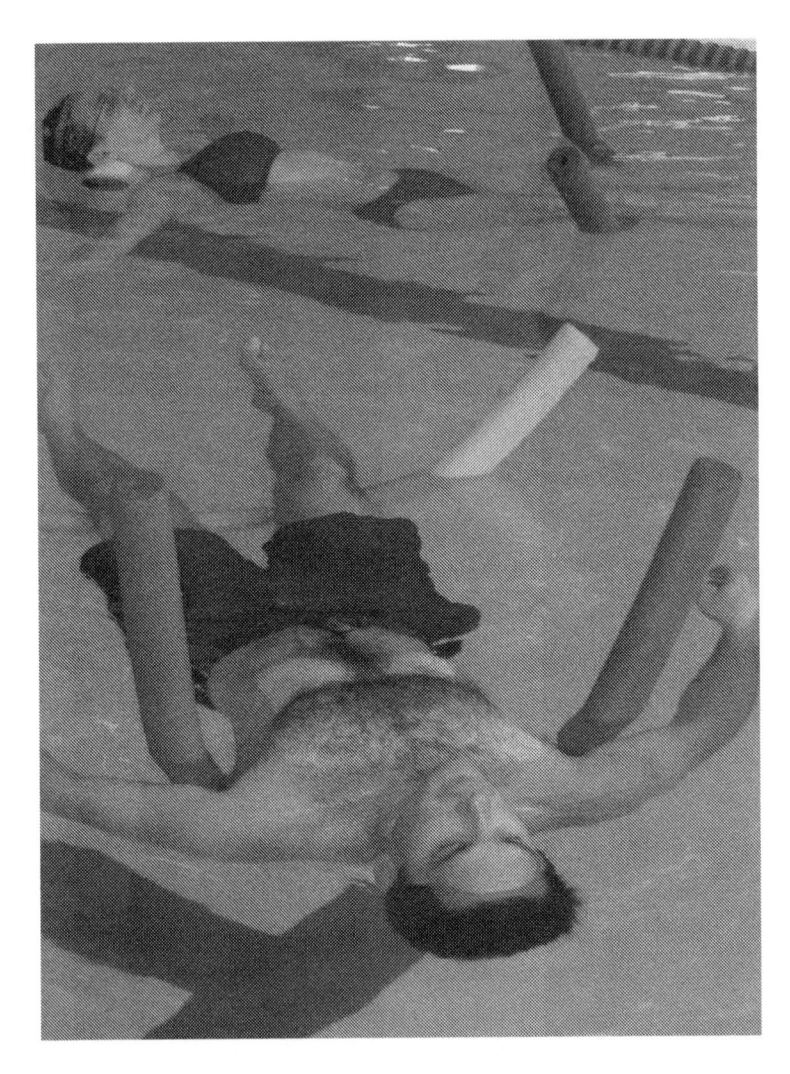

Resting Pose/Corpse

Providing the water is not cold, this can be a wonderful time to just relax and listen perhaps to some soothing music, or submerge ears under water and listen to the breath. A foam dumb bell can be used as a headrest. The heels can also rest on the pool deck or stairs. One noodle can be placed under the armpits and a second one under the knees. If the student needs assistance, it is a good time for the instructor to get into the pool and help them. Keep inner body nice and soft and surrender. Stay here for as long as you like.

MORE ADVANCED WORK

-This is **not** appropriate for a general class, but individuals may want to explore this area by themselves.
-If students have good body awareness, and experience of yoga already; this can be a wonderful time to try and move forwards in some areas that elude them on land.

24- Handstand

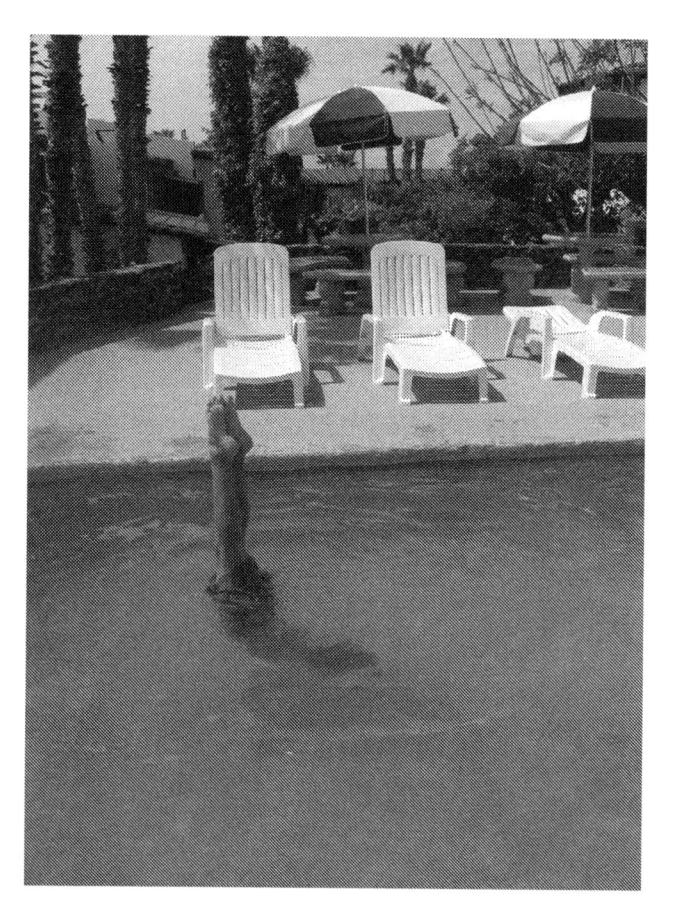

KEY STUDENT INSTRUCTIONS

-Retain breath as you bring hands to pool floor.
-Lift one leg, then the other as you push into hands.
-Keep legs together.
-Hold as long as comfortable.

Work in Asana or Variations:
-See how different the pose is by varying water depth.
-Walk hands along pool floor while keeping legs straight.
-Arch back into handstand. (I like a nose clip)
-Move from handstand into torpedo sculling.

POOLSIDE TEACHER NOTES

-Check for vertical legs.
-Keep floating ribs in.

The Bandhas or Locks

During the practice of asana and breath control, the yoga practitioner often engages muscular contractions that can help facilitate the ascent of life's energies within the more subtle body. I believe that we use them even more in the water, although maybe not cognizing that fact. These contractions are known as bandhas and there are three primary ones.

Important note

Awareness and initial practice of applying the bandhas should be learned by a yoga instructor and treated with great respect for them can move energies in an angular or balanced fashion.

The Three Bandhas are:
-Mula or root contraction
-Uddiyana or stomach contraction
-Jalandhara or chin lock.

My teacher explained it to me by imagining the lock system of a canal or inland waterway filling up in a contained area and elevating the boat to that level. The lock then opens and the boat moves along another section of the waterway.

Mula Bandha

Also known as root contraction, is best learned on land, but is used in combination with uddiyana bandha. It essentially prevents vital currents from flowing out of the body. It is the hardest of all three bandhas mentioned here because it is so subtle. A slight contraction of the anus is moving in the right direction and this is technically called aswini mudra.

Uddiyana Bandha

"Uddiyana", means "flying up", and it is used to cultivate the movement of ascending Prana, or life energies. The stomach muscles are pulled in slightly and then lifted up. A bit like when you catch a glimpse of yourself in the mirror and imagine what you would look like 10 pounds lighter... only still breathing. It lengthens the inner walls of the rib cage and frees the spine.

Typically whether you know it or not, the direction of asanas is to incorporate this inner lift. This transforms not only the physical body by allowing more energy into it, but the mind too. You can literally see the difference in a person's posture and attitude when they move about life subtly engaging this bandha.

Jalandhara Bandha

Also known as the chin lock, and is not looked at in great depth in this book, but worth mentioning as it is associated with the regulation and maintenance of the thyroid and parathyroid, and typically many students with problems in this area are attracted to water activity.

Keeping the length in the back of the neck, the chin drops down to the lifted chest. There are some poses that lend themselves very nicely to applying this lock, like for example a modified bridge pose or the noble seal pose, but even standing in Mountain pose, the chin lock can be applied. The breath should still flow unless you have received other training from your guru or yoga teacher.

25 – Torpedo Scull (engaging uddiyana bandha)

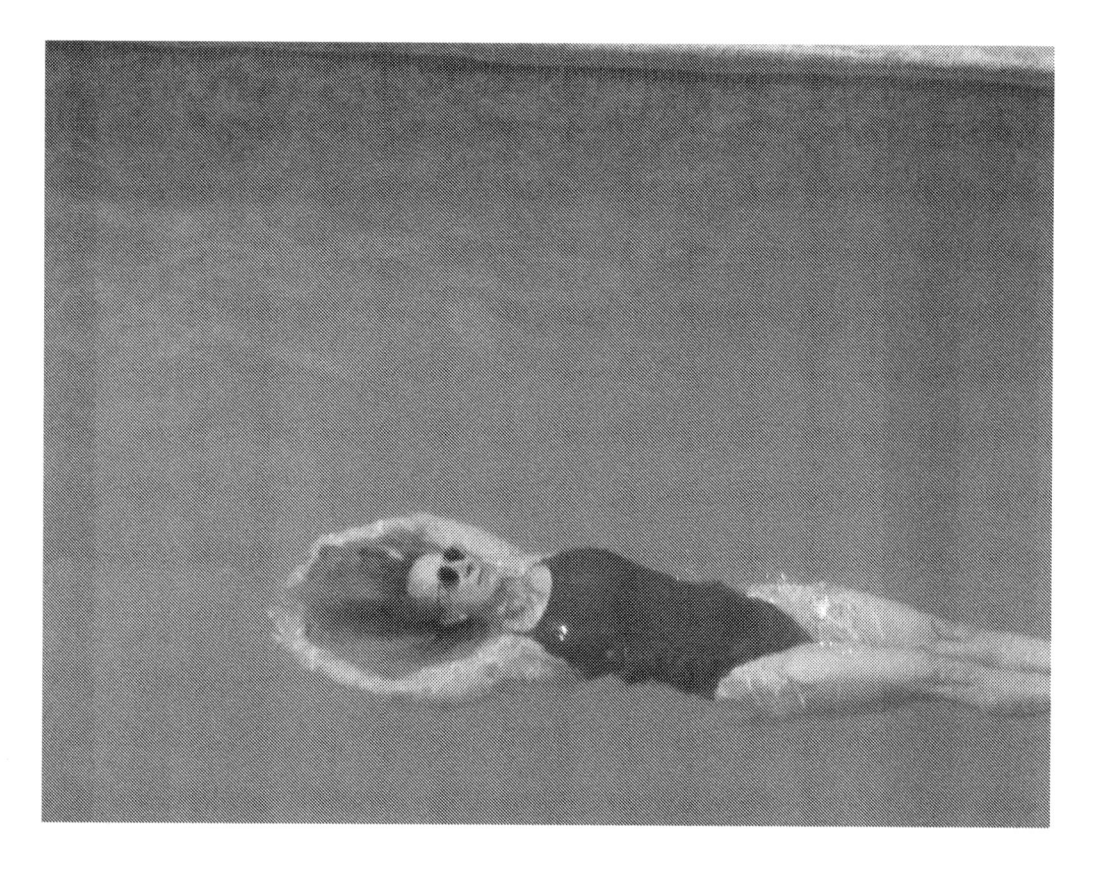

Torpedo

KEY STUDENT INSTRUCTIONS
-Lift both shins to water surface and point toes.
-Lift heart and straighten legs.
-Extend arms overhead palms facing wall behind.
-Open fingers and shake hands to travel across pool.
-Keep legs together and point toes.
-Draw belly and abdomen in and up.

Work in Asana or Variations:
-You can travel very fast in this pose.
-Make sure the breath is nice and even.
-Visualize drawing in, and retaining more oxygen and Prana.

POOLSIDE TEACHER NOTES
-Move hands in crescent moons fingers together.
-Thighs and hips push up.
-Chest open.

26 – Reverse Torpedo

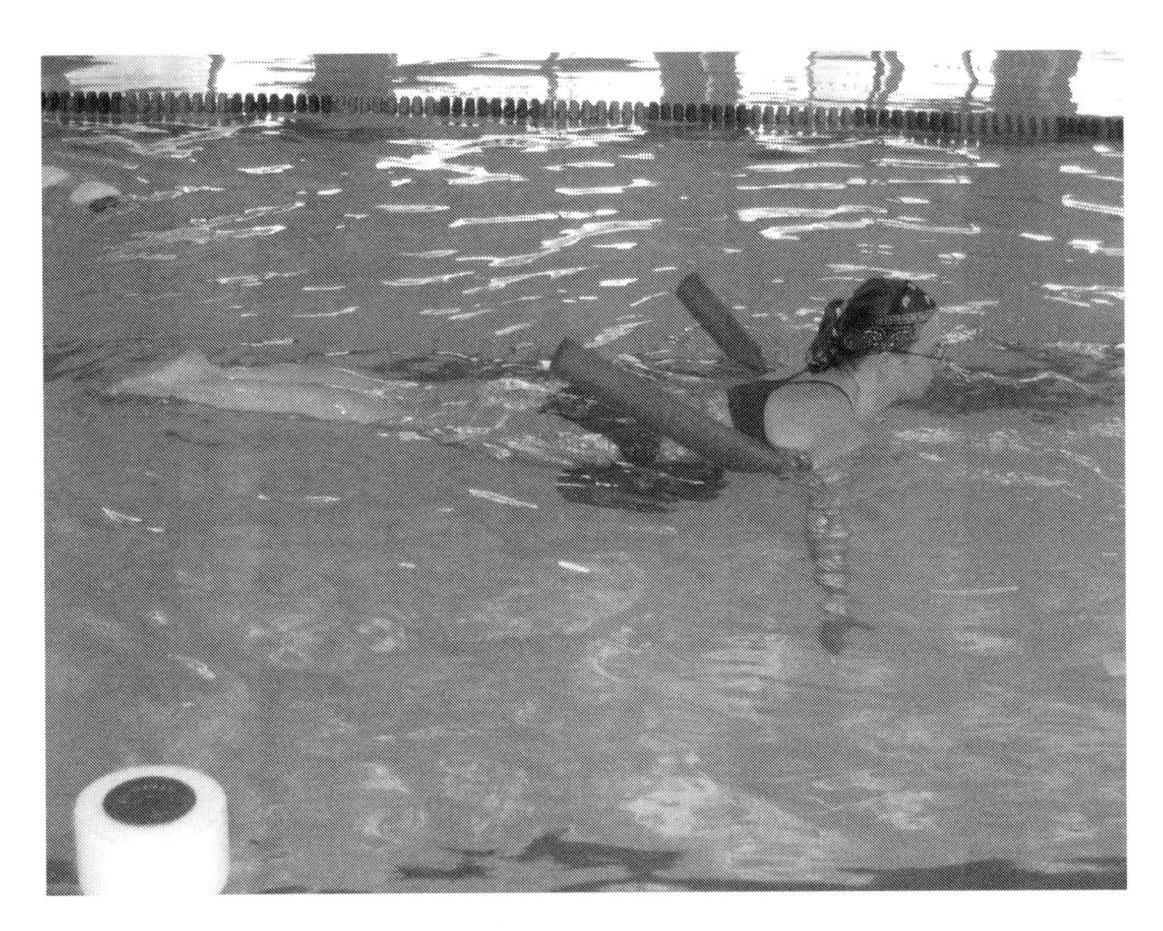

Reverse Torpedo

This is a little harder to sustain for as long, but it works the back, arms and legs nicely and is good for focusing on the exhale especially. It can be done with a noodle initially.

KEY STUDENT INSTRUCTIONS

-Take noodle across upper chest and under armpits.
-Lift both legs behind and keep straight
-Keep fingers together and "scull" hands in anti-clockwise circle to propel feet first.

POOLSIDE TEACHER NOTES

-Fully engage uddiyana bandha
-Press legs together.
-Lift head and heart.

26. Reverse Torpedo

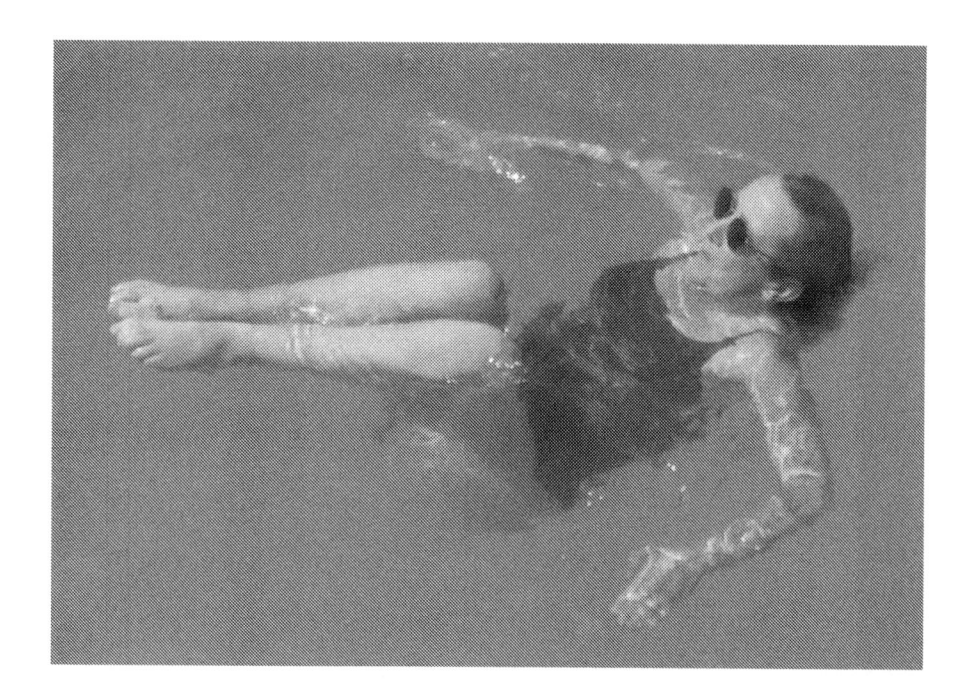

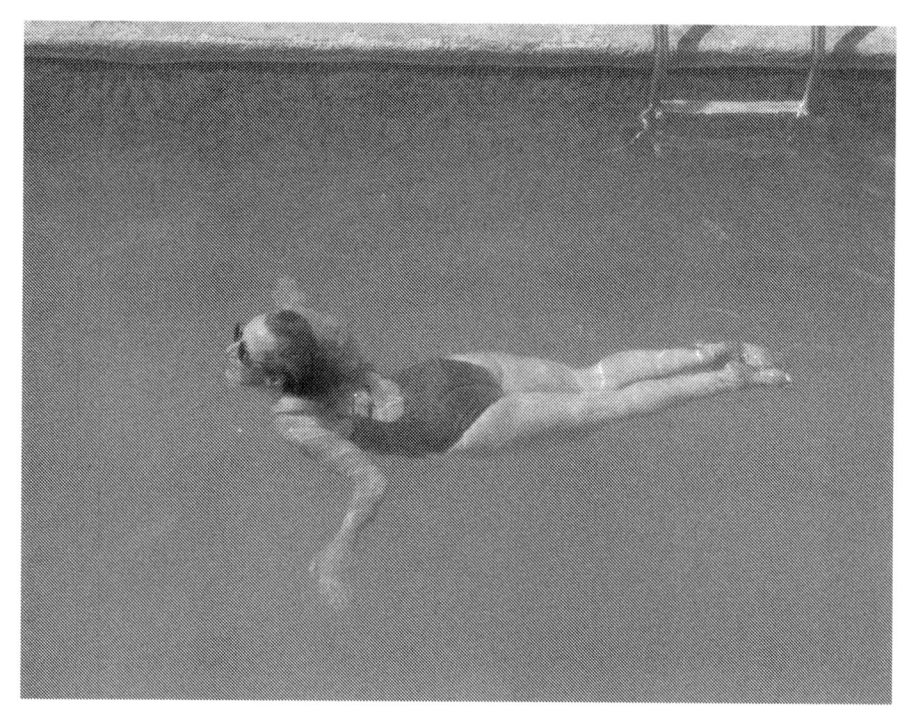

Work in Asana or Variations:
-Great tummy toner to move from chest up, to chest down position by sculling the hands.
-Figures of eight in hand movement with chest up and circles and push with hands to take legs back.
-Coordinate with breath or hold each posture for a few breaths.
-Keep shoulders down, and draw Half Moon with hands keeping fingers tight together.

27- Poolside Arm Balance

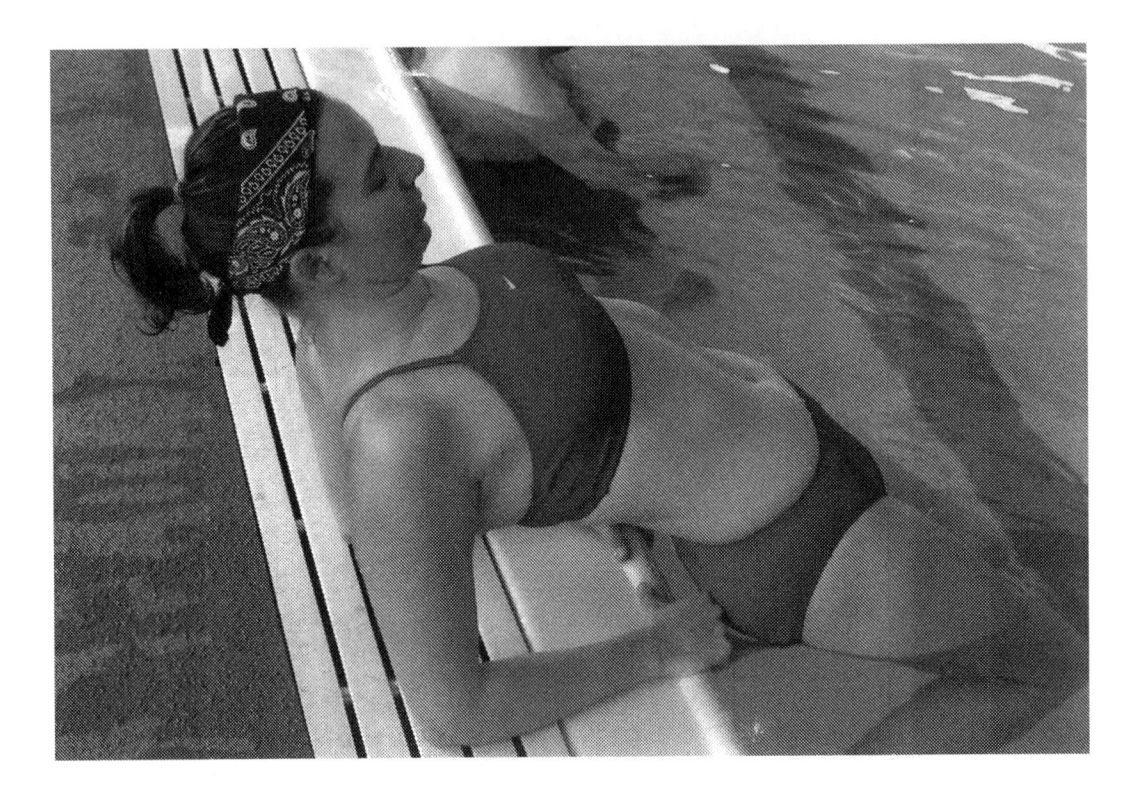

27. Poolside Arm Balance

KEY STUDENT INSTRUCTIONS

-Face to middle pool and using arms lift torso out of the water and rest on forearms.
-Bring soles of feet to wall and push hips forward.
-Draw organs into the back body

Work in Asana or Variations:
-Try resting buttocks to wall and then raising both legs keeping them straight.
-Could extend front of neck and look up instead of having the chin lock.

POOLSIDE TEACHER NOTES

-Try to get elbows under shoulders.
-Lift heart.
-Keep thighs parallel.

28- Chakric Wheel

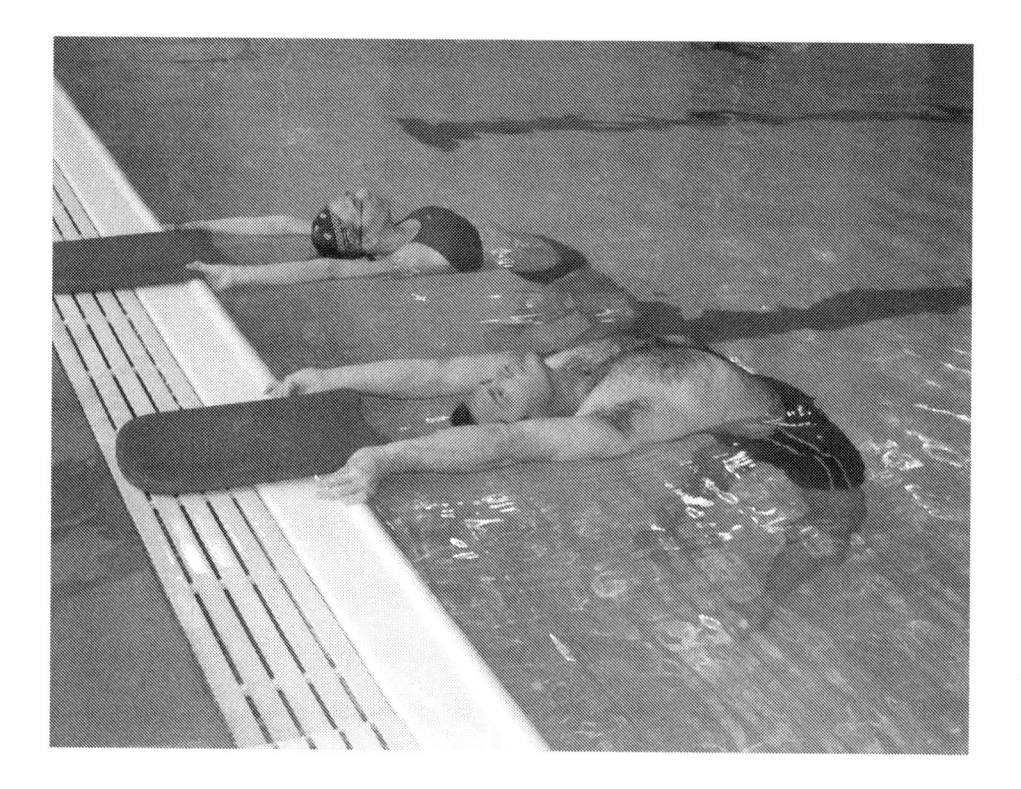

28. Chakric Wheel

KEY STUDENT INSTRUCTIONS

-Stand away from wall feet hip distance apart.
-Push hips forward, and look up.
-Reach hands to wall behind.
-Hold on to wall, or use a float.
-Keep toes facing forward and push into floor.

Work in Asana or Variations:
-In deeper water can rest base of skull to deck, take arms back in the same way and hold on.
-Push down with feet and straighten legs.
-Lift heart, and take head back.
-Keep elbows in.

POOLSIDE TEACHER NOTES

-The float helps to space hands and deepen armpits.
-Broaden upper back.

29- Monkey Stretch

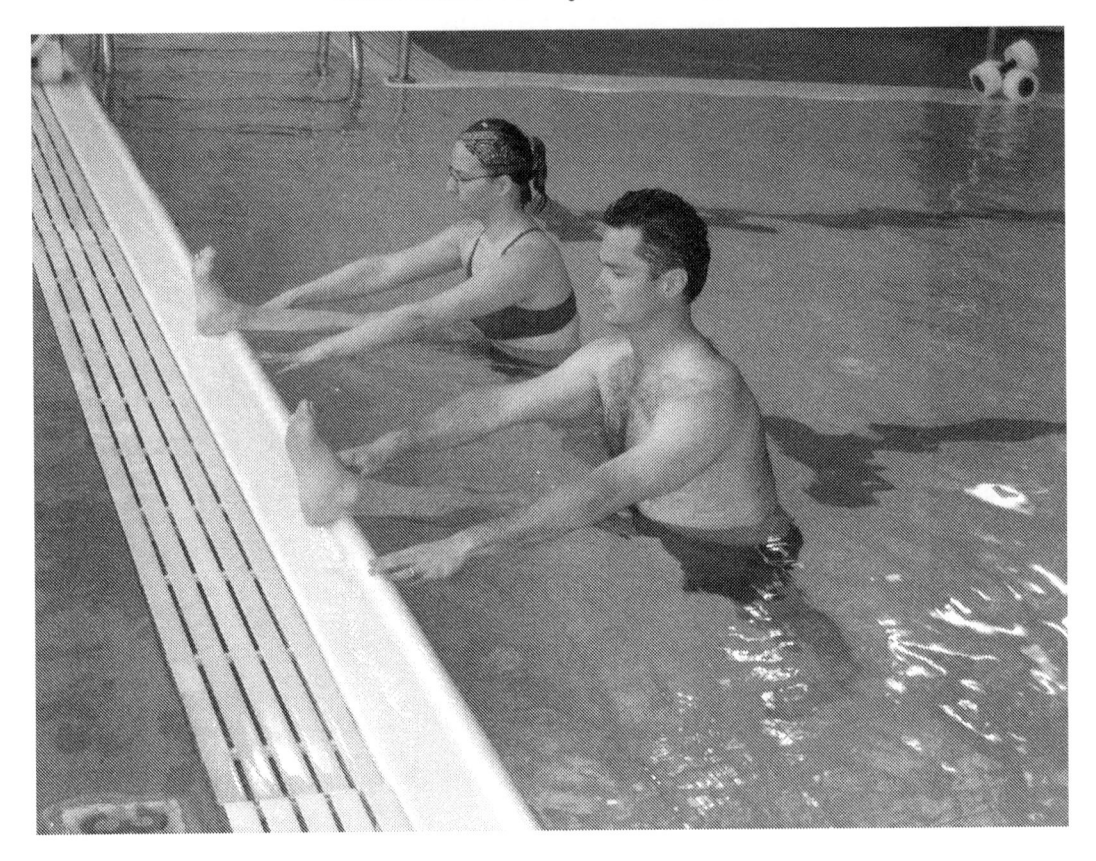

29. Monkey Stretch. **Be careful** not to hyper extend the knee joint.

KEY STUDENT INSTRUCTIONS

-Stand on Left leg, raise Right leg and put heel on pool deck.
-Keep hips level.
-Lengthen spine and ease bones of legs back to muscles.
-Keep supporting leg strong.

POOLSIDE TEACHER NOTES

-Need to find correct depth.
-Do not force this.

Work in Asana or Variations:

-If legs o.k., try taking arms overhead, palms facing each other.
-If in wading style pool you can sink down into the pose and bring finger tips to pool floor.
-Front heel could also rest on pool step.

30- Deep Twist with Shoulder Stability

Remember, not suitable for pregnant ladies.

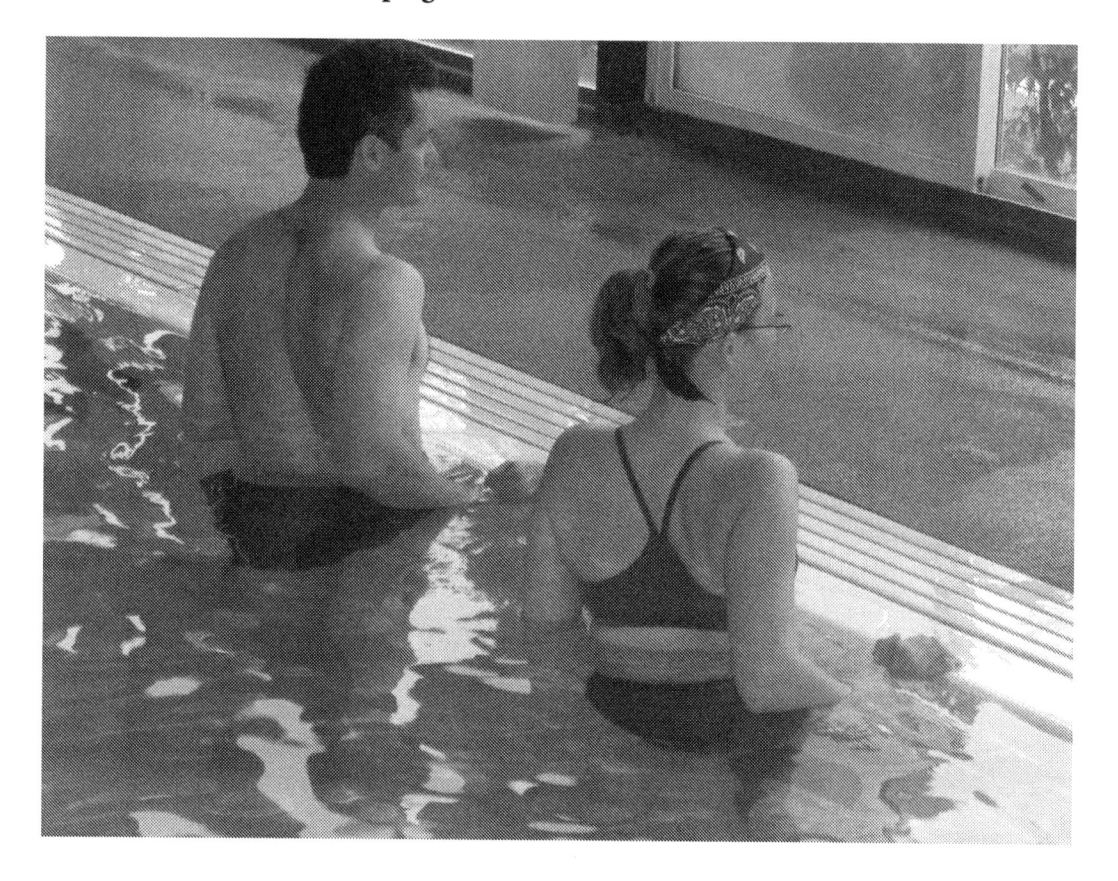

Deep Twist and Shoulder Stability

KEY STUDENT INSTRUCTIONS

-Stand with Right hip to pool wall.
-Step Right foot forward and keep both legs straight.
-Rotate belly to Right and bring hands to the wall.
-Keep elbows in and shoulders down.
-Repeat on the other side

POOLSIDE TEACHER NOTES

-Push back heel down.
-Keep inner body soft.
-Lengthen neck.

Work in Asana or Variations:
-Stand closer to wall.
-Bend Right leg and rest outer thigh to wall.
-Rotate belly to wall and extend arms along deck.
-Try facing palms hands up to broaden upper back.

31- Reverse Triangle Pose

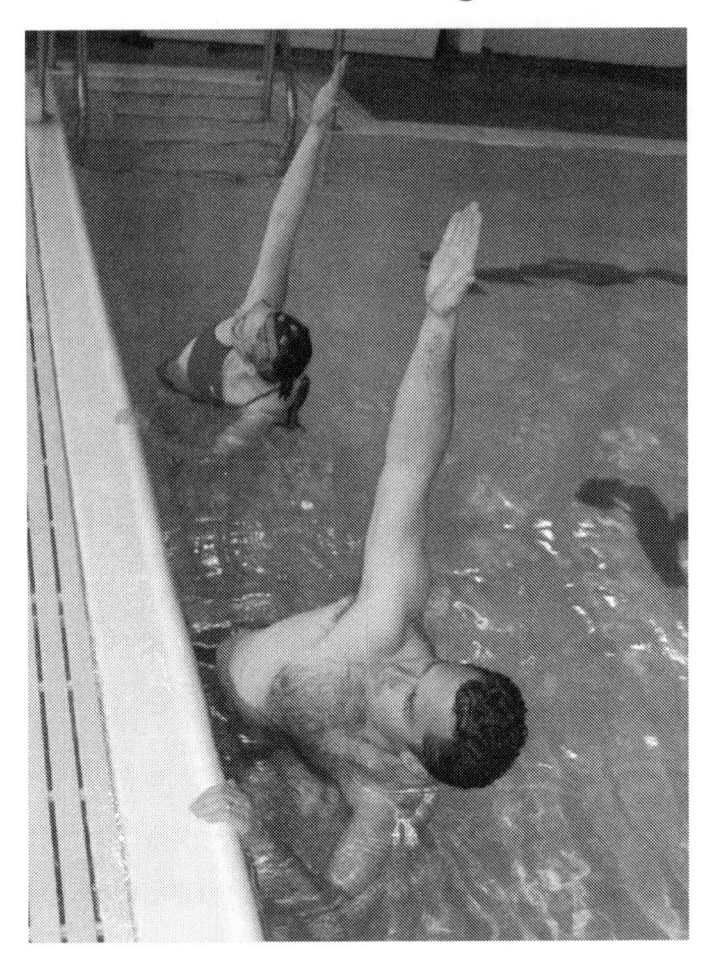

Reverse Triangle

KEY STUDENT INSTRUCTIONS

-Stand with Right hip close to wall.
-Step Left leg back.
-Lengthen Left side of torso and rotate belly to Right.
-Hold on to pool wall with Left hand.
-Extend Right arm overhead.
-Repeat to Left side.

Work in Asana or Variations:
-If space behind:
-Try lifting Left leg.
-Push heel out
-Work torso to pool wall.

POOLSIDE TEACHER NOTES

-Push Left heel into floor.
-Breathe into Left kidney.
-Spine and neck long.
-Stack shoulders.

32- Pelvic Tilt & Feet to Wall (Cat-Cow Variation)

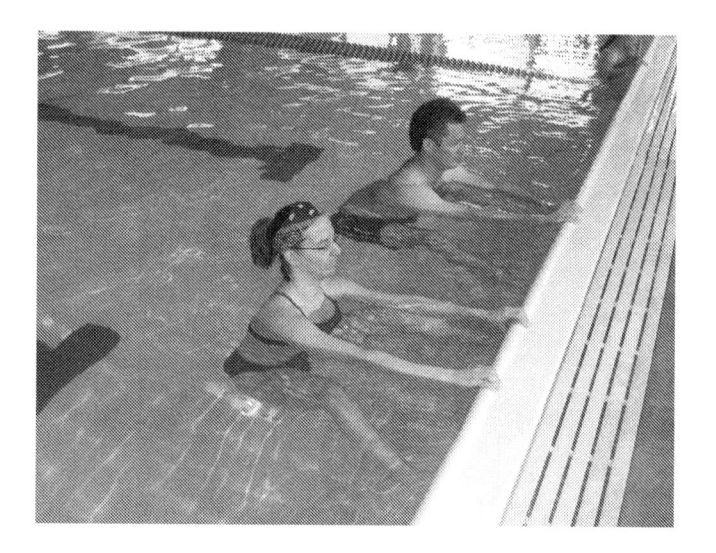

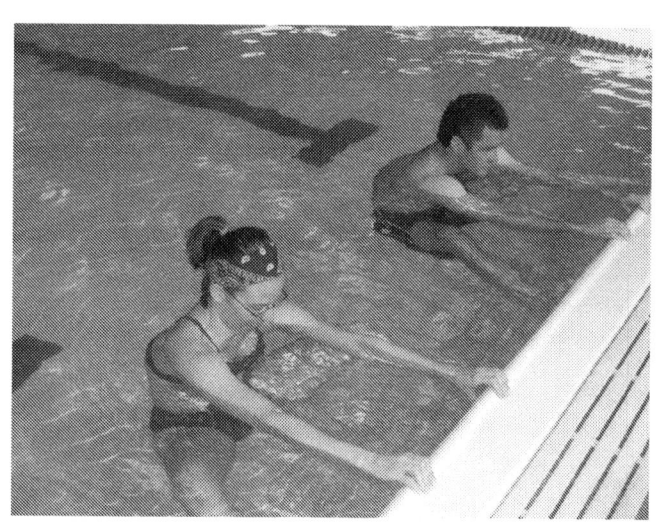

Cat/Cow Variation

KEY STUDENT INSTRUCTIONS

-Face wall and hold onto edge with hands.
-Step Right foot to wall, wider than the hip.
-Step Left foot to wall, wider than the hip.
-Exhale and round back. Tuck tailbone under.
-Inhale and lift chest and sit bones and look forward.
-Repeat a few times coordinating breath and movement.

Work in Asana or Variations:
-Try straightening legs on inhale.
-Keep lift in heart and shoulders down.

POOLSIDE TEACHER NOTES

-Toes face up to ceiling.
-Maintain shoulder stability.

33- Warrior 3 (Top Picture) & Backbend Scull (Bottom Picture)

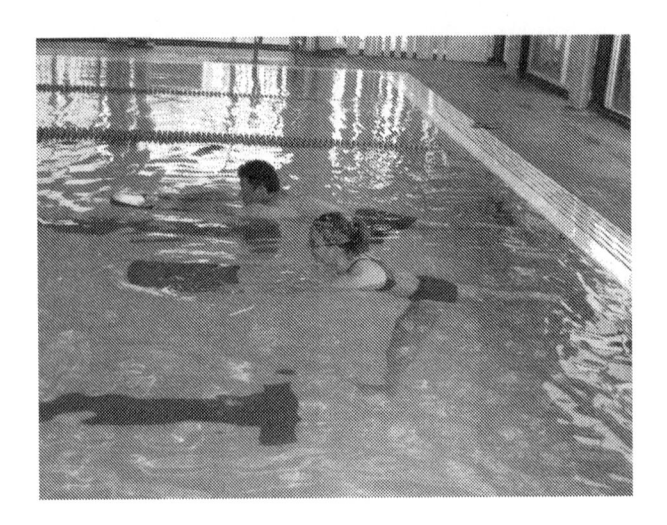

33. Warrior 3

KEY STUDENT INSTRUCTIONS

-Stand away from pool facing to center of pool.
-Raise Right leg behind and push sole of foot to wall.
-Use kick board and extend arms forward
-Lift heart
-Repeat to other side.

POOLSIDE TEACHER NOTES

-Both legs straight
-Shoulders down.

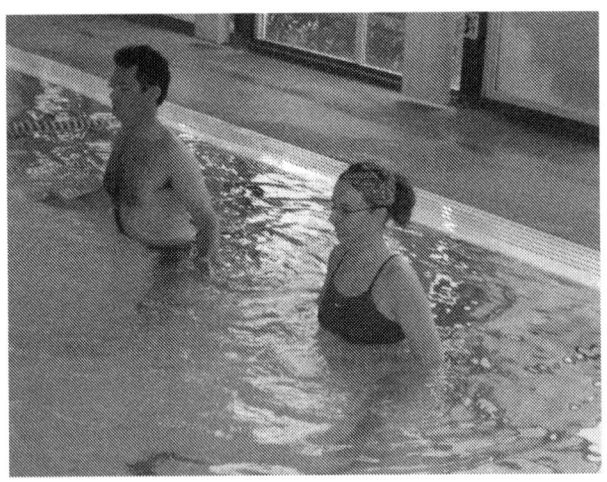

Backbend scull

Work in Asana or Variations:
-Loose the board, arch the back and draw little inward circles with hands.
-Push water away from you to keep Right foot in contact with wall.

34- Hip Opener & Side Bend

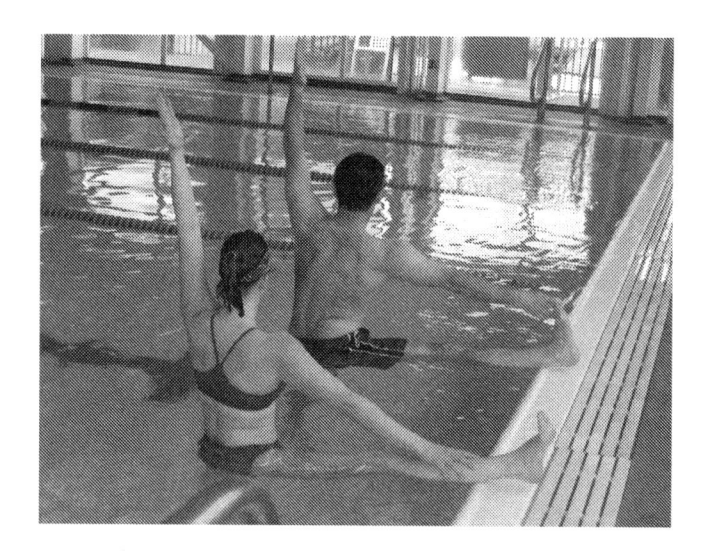

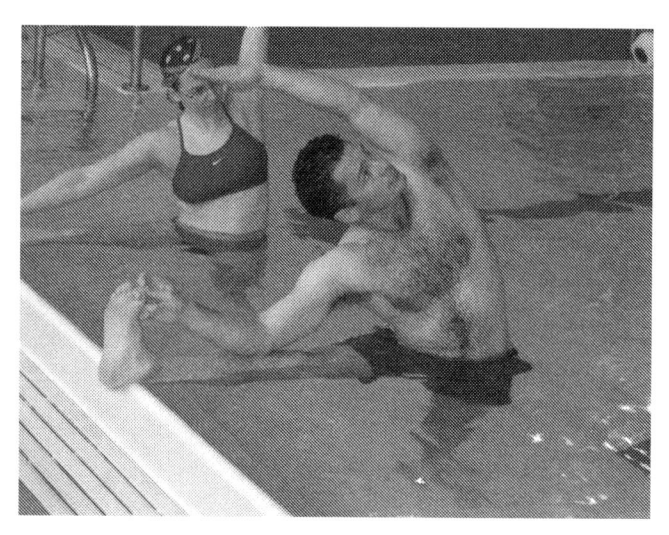

Hip Opener and Side bend

KEY STUDENT INSTRUCTIONS

-Stand with Right hip facing wall.
-Open up in hip.
-Rest Right heel to deck or sole Right foot to wall.
-Hold big Right toe with Right hand if accessible.
-Extend Left arm overhead.
-Repeat to Left side.

POOLSIDE TEACHER NOTES

-Keep hips level.
-May hold on anywhere on Right leg.
-Palm facing Right.
-Armpits deep.

Work in Asana or Variations:

-Keep chest facing forward and extend Left arm overhead close to ear.
-Close armpit.
-Lengthen Right side torso.

35-Basic Sun Salutations

One can adapt Sun Salutations to suit whatever environment you find yourself in, such as an airplane or sitting in a chair, or even lying down, and being in the water is only another type of environment that can embrace this lovely dance of asanas. As with the individual asanas that make up the sequence, it is best not to go so deep in the water that you cannot deepen the groins or bend forwards a reasonable amount without putting the face under water.

I think it best to hold each of the asanas for a few breaths rather than an inhale or an exhale only as the water will become very choppy and disturb the mind too much.

A basic sequence of Sun Salutation could include: *(pictures on following pages)*

1. Standing Mountain, not too close to the wall.
2. Take arms overhead and hips forward in direction of a backbend. (optional)
3. Sit back into an imaginary chair, bending the knees with arms overhead. Have palms facing each other.
4. Step Right foot forward and bend knee to a lunge, Arms overhead. Left leg back and up on toes.
5. Step Right leg back to meet Left leg in Plank pose.
6. Bring forearms to wall keeping elbows in.
7. Arch back into Up Dog.
8. Push hips back to half forward bend position. (Torso lengthening pose)
9. Step Right leg forward to lunge. Arms overhead. Have palms facing each other.
10. Step Left leg forward into chair position. Have both arms overhead.
11. Stand in arm overhead pose and push hips fwd in direction of a back bend.
12. Bring hands together in "Namaste", prayer position across the heart.

Variations:

-Placing sole of Right foot to wall in lunge rather than to floor.
-Warrior 2 could be added to open hip joint.
-A standing twist from a lunge could be added.

The variations are endless. Just remember to try doing the same amount of repetitions on both sides, and don't forget to breathe.

For students new to yoga, it may be difficult for them to follow verbal instructions or even hear what you are trying to say. Keep it simple. It's a good way to occupy the mind, and give it something to focus on. With the practice of concentration, body awareness and control of the breath can improve. Just like on land, it is an area where you will have some creative fun in.

Basic Sun Salutations

<u>Sun Salutations</u>

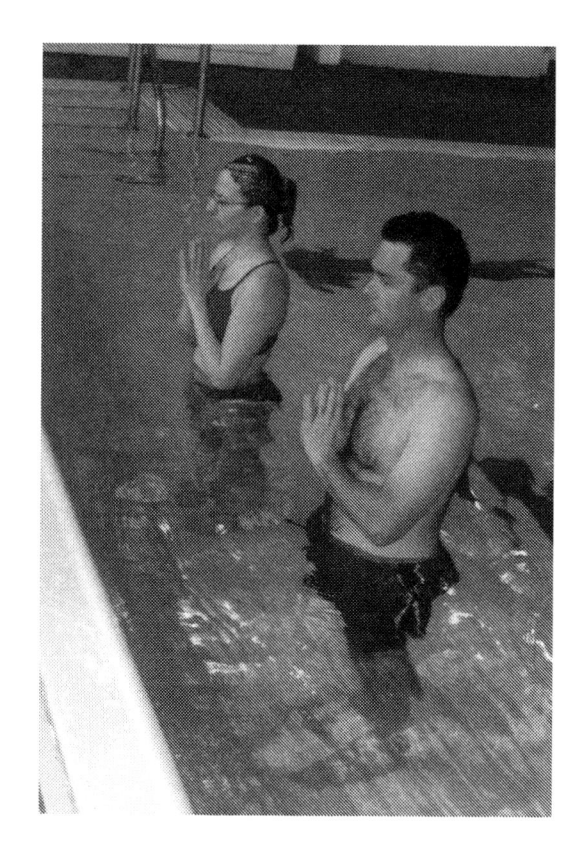

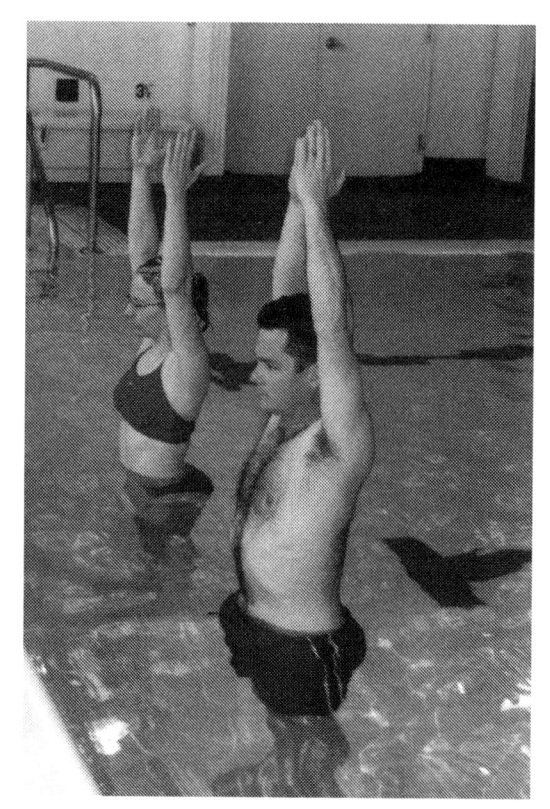

1- Standing Mountain Pose   2- Arms Overhead Pose

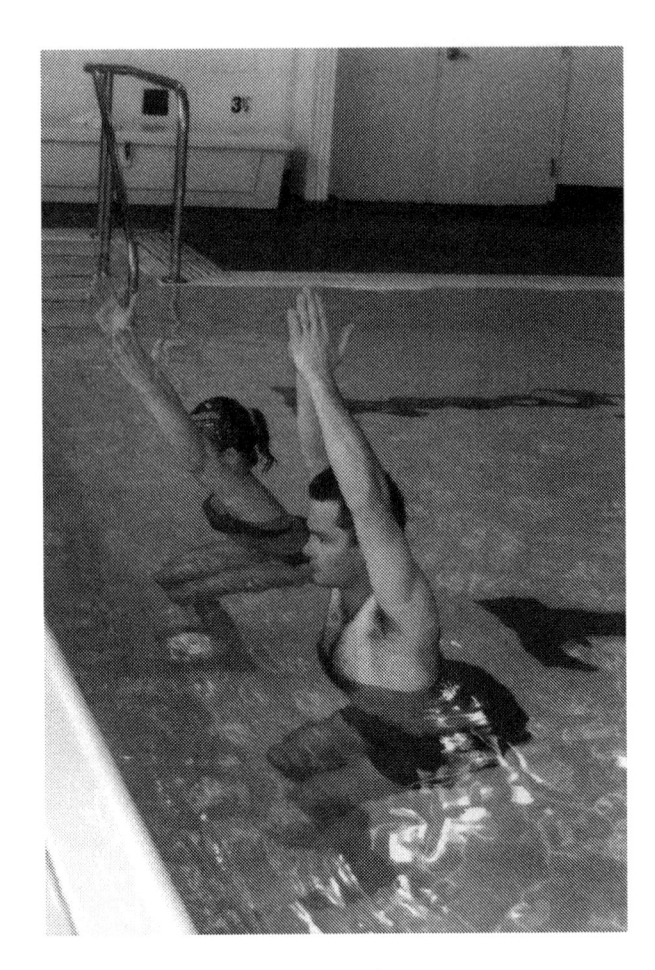

3- Imaginary Chair Pose

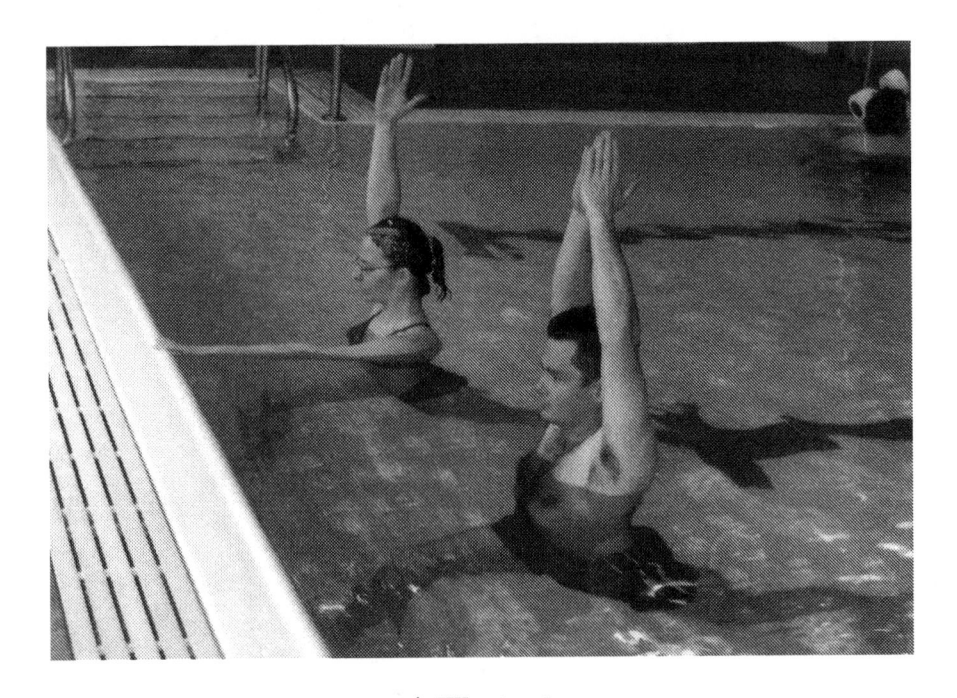

4- Warrior 1

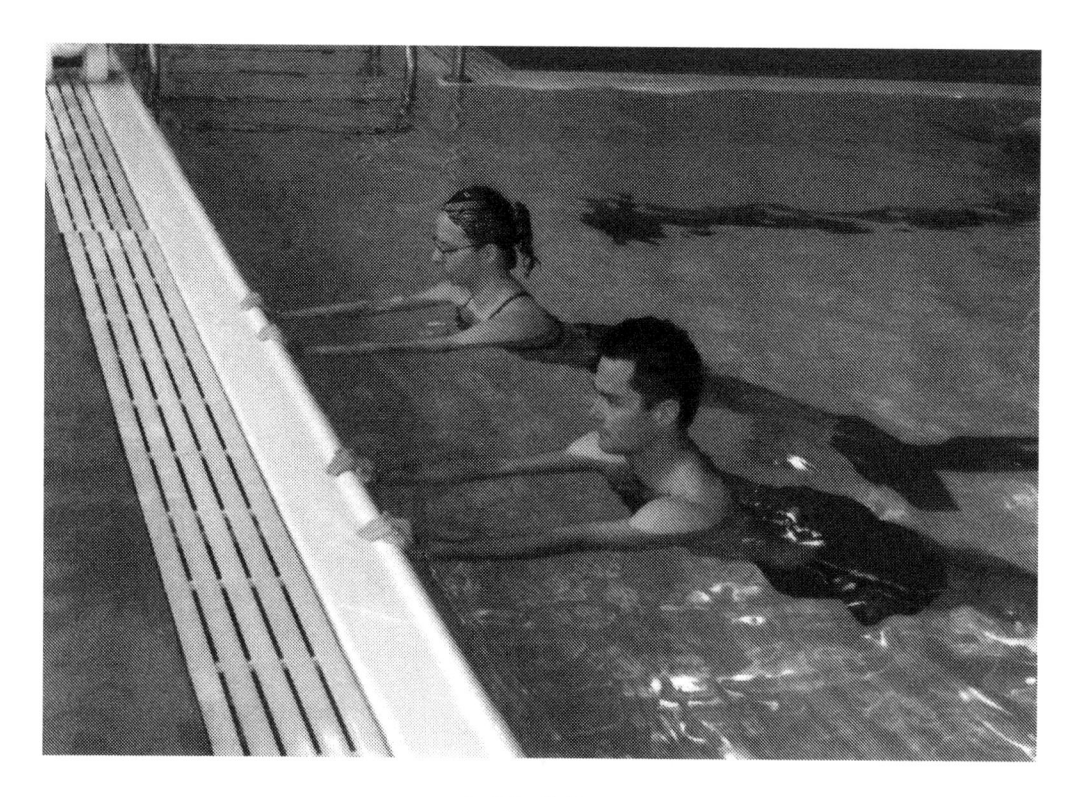

5- Plank Pose

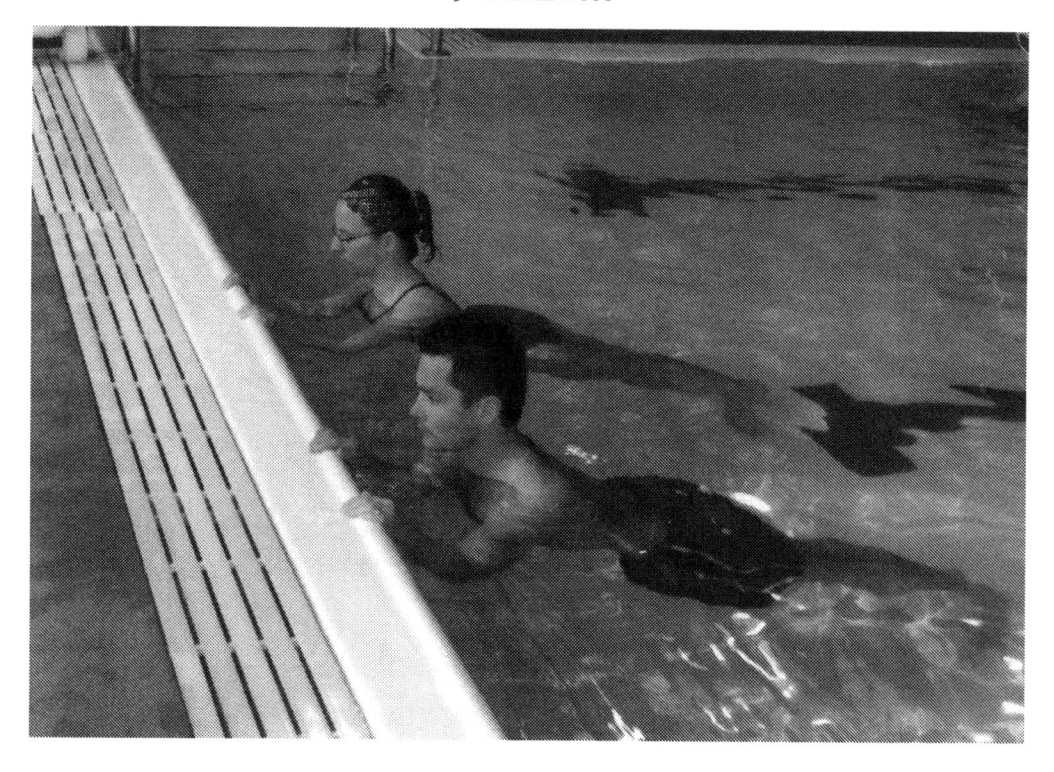

6- Forearms at the wall

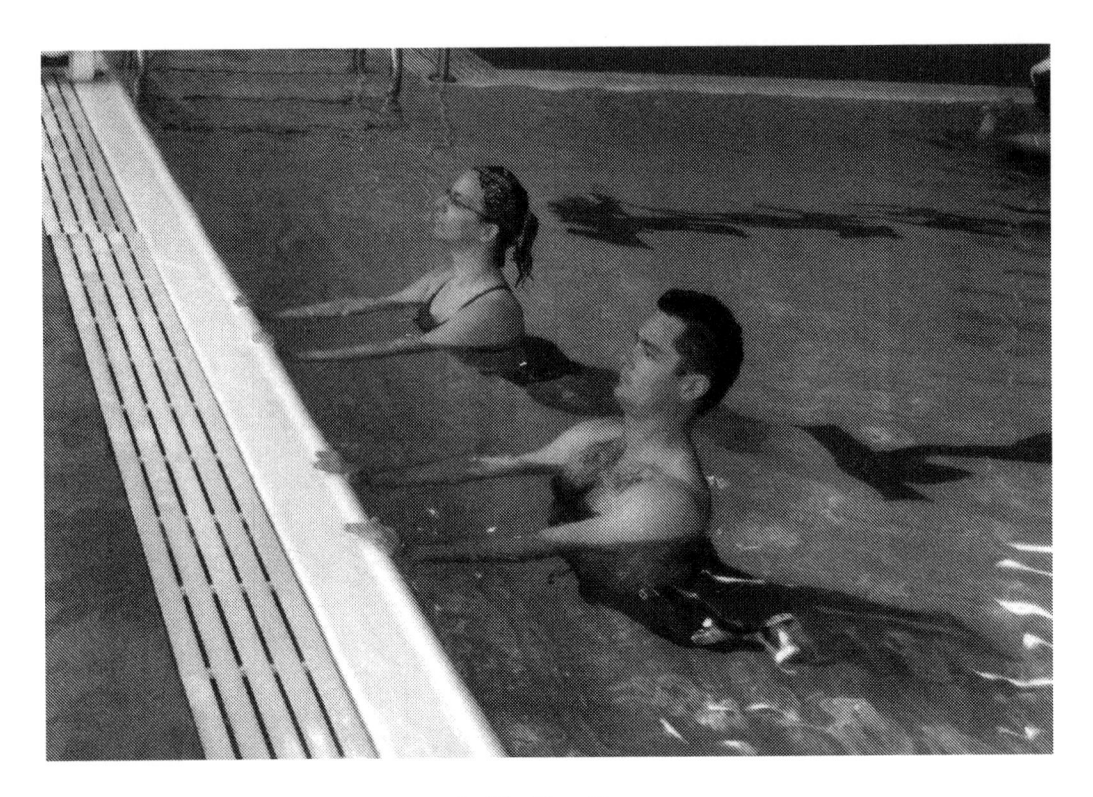

7- Up Dog Pose

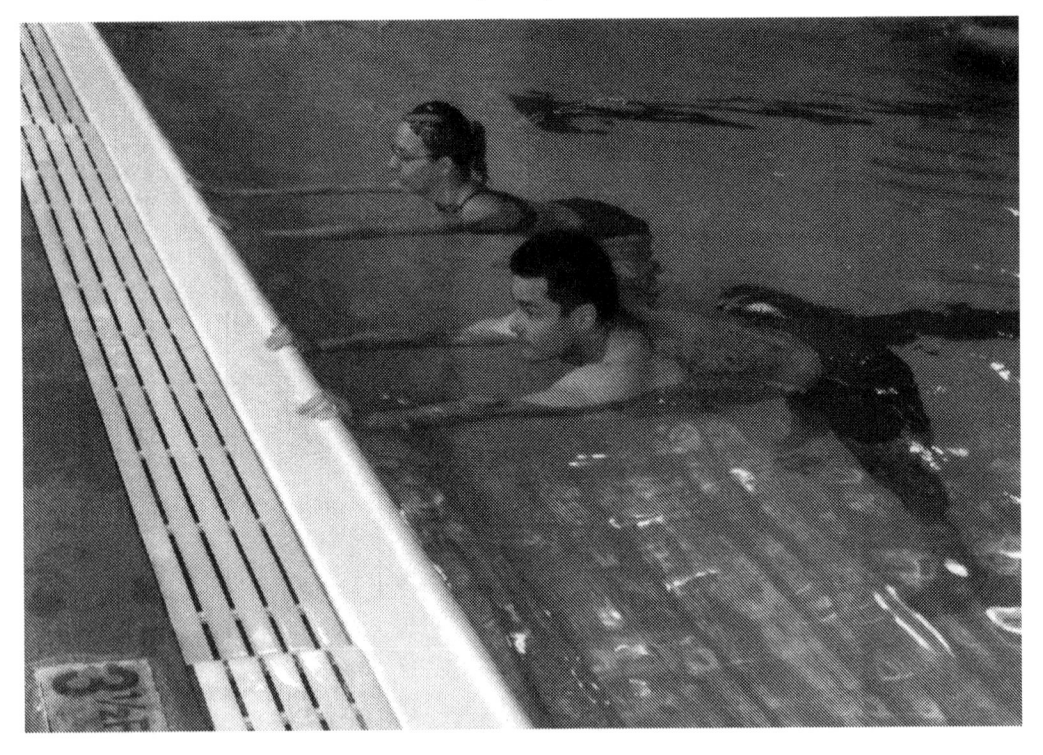

8 - Torso Lengthening Pose

"BE LIKE THE WATER MAKING IT'S WAY THROUGH THE CRACKS. DO NOT BE ASSERTIVE, BUT ADJUST TO THE OBJECT, AND YOU SHALL FIND A WAY ROUND OR THROUGH IT. IF NOTHING WITHIN YOU STAYS RIGID, OUTWARD THINGS WILL DISCLOSE THEMSELVES."

BRUCE LEE

Aqua Yoga and the Pre-Natal Student

"Ladies in waiting", can benefit from practicing Aqua Yoga, particularly if they are feeling heavy and lacking in vitality. Not only can they become seemingly weightless, they can move around in the same medium as their baby, which can be another important symbolic bond between the two. Very often, the modern pregnant woman has to work into late pregnancy whilst still maintaining the home, and or caring for other children. She can therefore be under a great amount of stress at this time. That, coupled with the increase in body weight can make them feel miserable, undesirable, and unable to cope with life and their changing bodies. It is very important that the mother minimizes any negative emotionality at this time, as her level of consciousness will have an affect on the baby, (we all affect one another) To the baby, she is the totality of his/her perceivable universe, and the mothers thoughts, words, and actions interrelating with other people, will greatly affect the predisposition of the child in, or out of her womb.

1 loved floating in the water with my ears under the water, which is not suitable for everyone, where the inner sounds can be heard as the mind slows down. For the experienced student, it is a wonderful way to explore the first level of sense withdrawal through the ears without using the thumbs. Swimming under water if it is possible, is also very profound.

I was fortunate to deliver my first child in a water birthing pool, and it was a positive experience for us both. For me, the warm water did a lot to relieve my anxiety, lower back pain, and therefore allowed me to think more clearly. I could change my erratic breathing patterning which I was unaware of before. For my son, it meant a wondrous, familiar transition into an alien environment. He came out smiling, and for the most part always has a smile on his face. Françoise Freedman has a book out for pregnancy, which you might want to look at for some gentle water stretches.

Some seasoned yoga students prefer to take their land yoga practice into the water, especially near the end of their term when one can feel heavy and confined literally. Coincidentally, the chakra at the tailbone known as muladhara is linked to the Saturn state of consciousness where one can feel limited or confined. It is known as an Earth element and when a woman is pregnant, the natural instinct is to get down to the earth and squat as they do in simpler civilizations that attune to nature better than we do. Practicing the hip openers benefits the mother physically as she opens up for the birth, but also mystically, as the sacral area relates to the Water element known as Jupiter. It is linked to expansion, which they can relate to physically, but is also an ascension psychologically, from confinements of the mind and its fearful thoughts. Just being surrounded by water, therefore can benefit the mothers on a deep, subconscious level.

Generally, I find that pregnant ladies can do pretty much the same as other students, but need to be wary of deep visceral twists. A twist in the upper back can feel nice though, and help with upper back discomfort. They can modify twisting poses to just activate movement in the upper spine. Backbends are not generally necessary on land, because the mother is usually gripping the inner body towards this bias even though it may be on a subtle level. In the water, being supported by water, some students who have had a strong practice on land like the alternate arm raising back bend described in the asana section. This is because they can sustain length and support in the front and back of the body in the water, whereas on land it is more difficult with the extra weight of the pregnancy. Even then, they only do very gentle backbends with strong legs. Even gentle backbends are probably best avoided unless the student has sound advise from her practitioner that it is o.k. to do so, and should not be-done-after the first trimester, as the baby's well being may be compromised.

If the student suffers from any discomfort in the legs or ankles, this too can be alleviated in the water. A regular practice can also help to avoid varicose veins. Extra time floating in the pool can be a beautiful time for mother and baby if the water temperature is conducive to that. A foam noodle under the armpits/knees and maybe the neck, cradles them both well, and gives the mother a chance to let go physically and mentally.

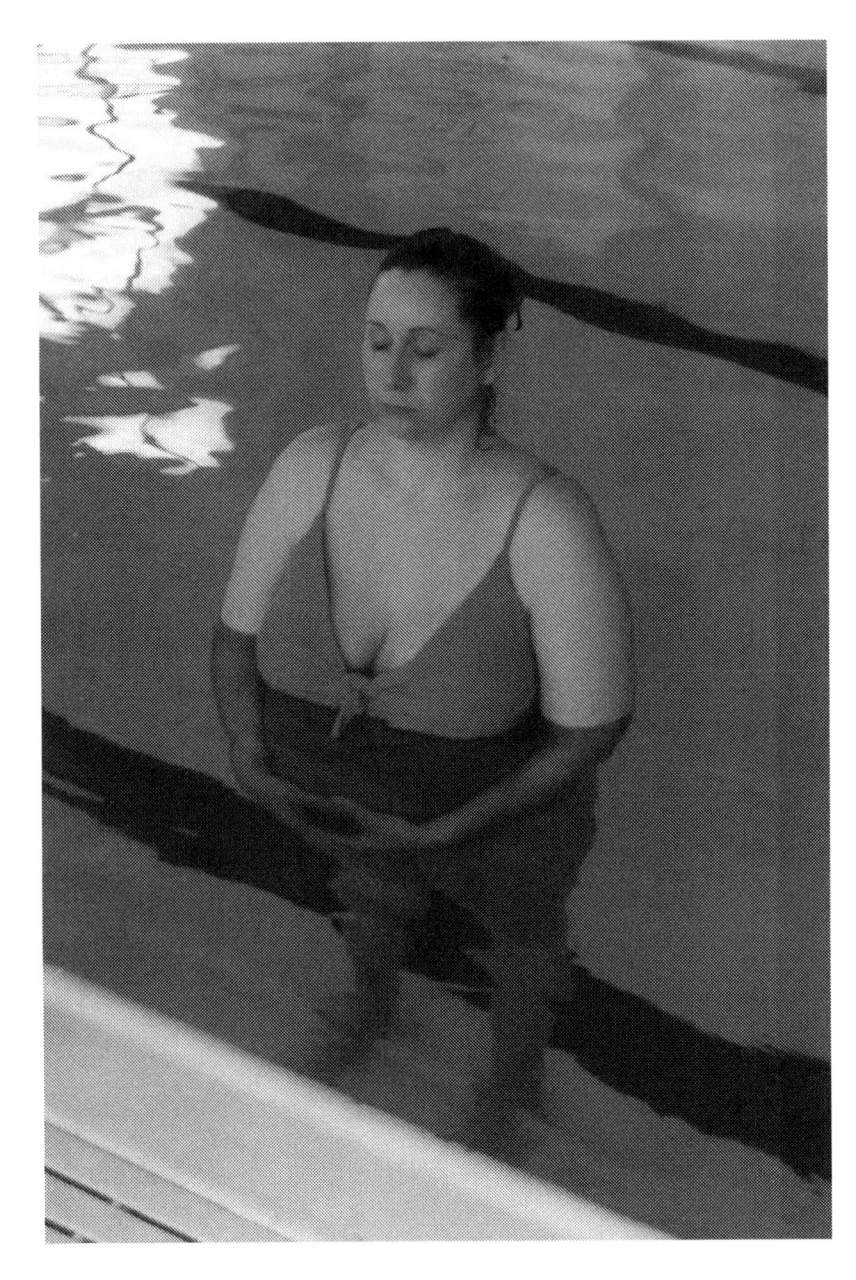

Serenity obtained amongst the confusion of body and mind changes.

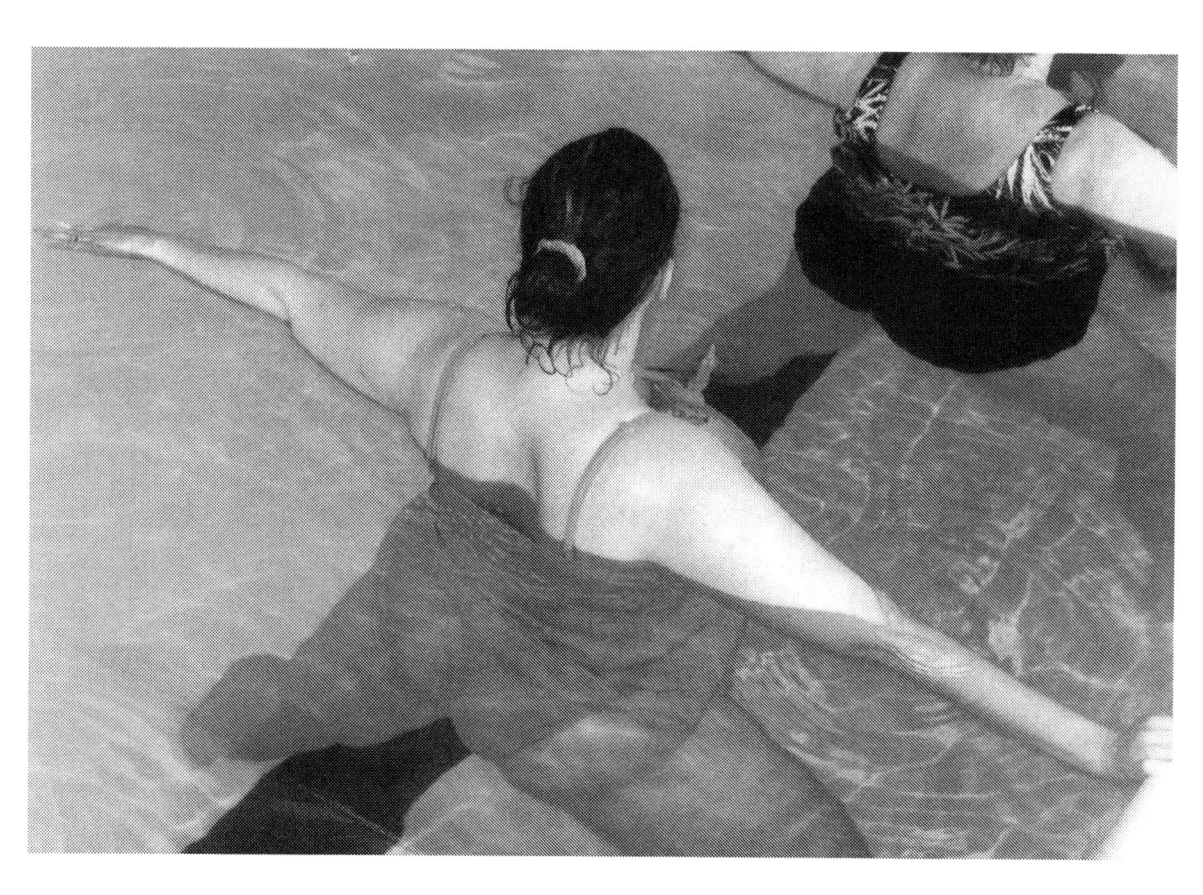

More space laterally for mother and baby in Warrior 2

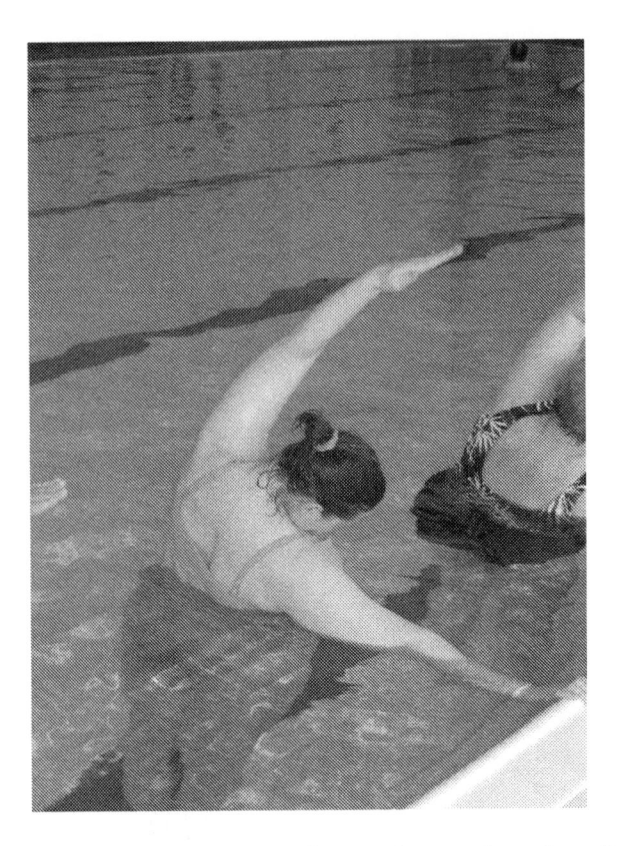

Nice side bend to open up, strengthen and tone the sides of the body

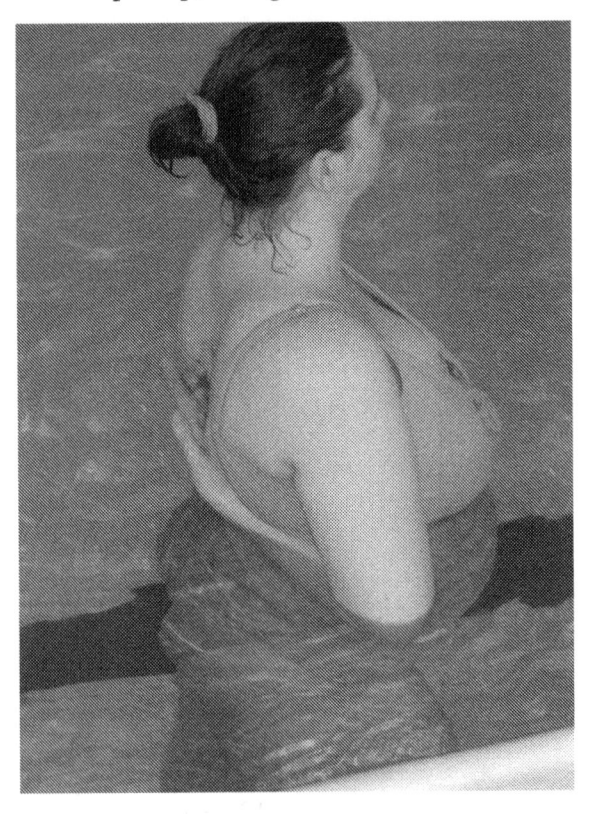

Posture can suffer as weight is gained, so shoulder work can be wonderful.

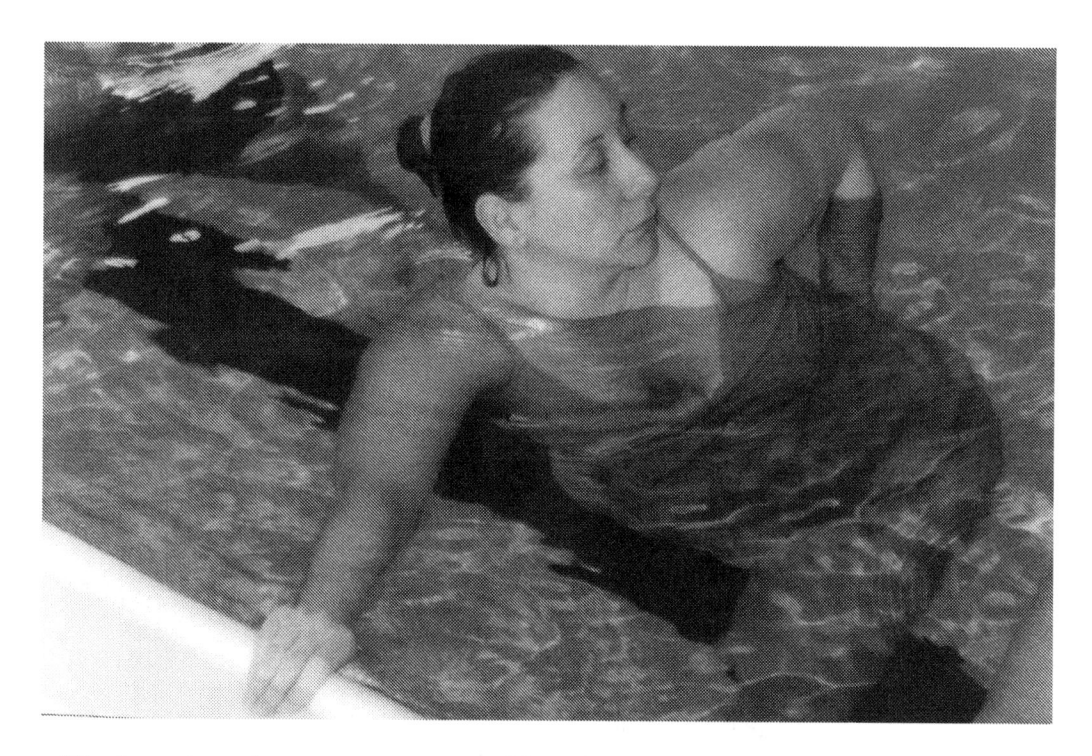

No deep visceral twists recommended but the upper spine still enjoys stimulation

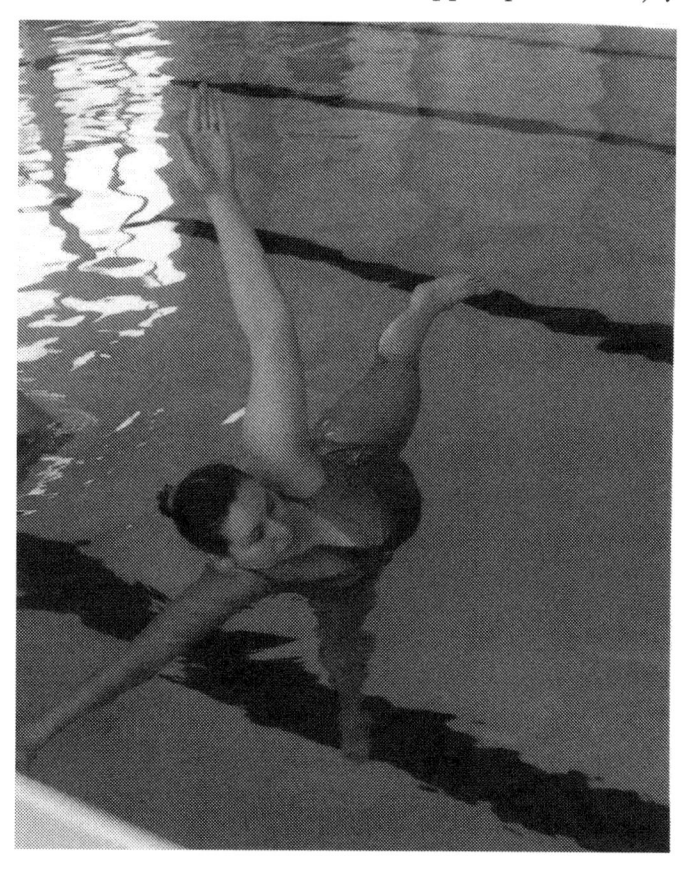

AH ! I can feel light and open my body !

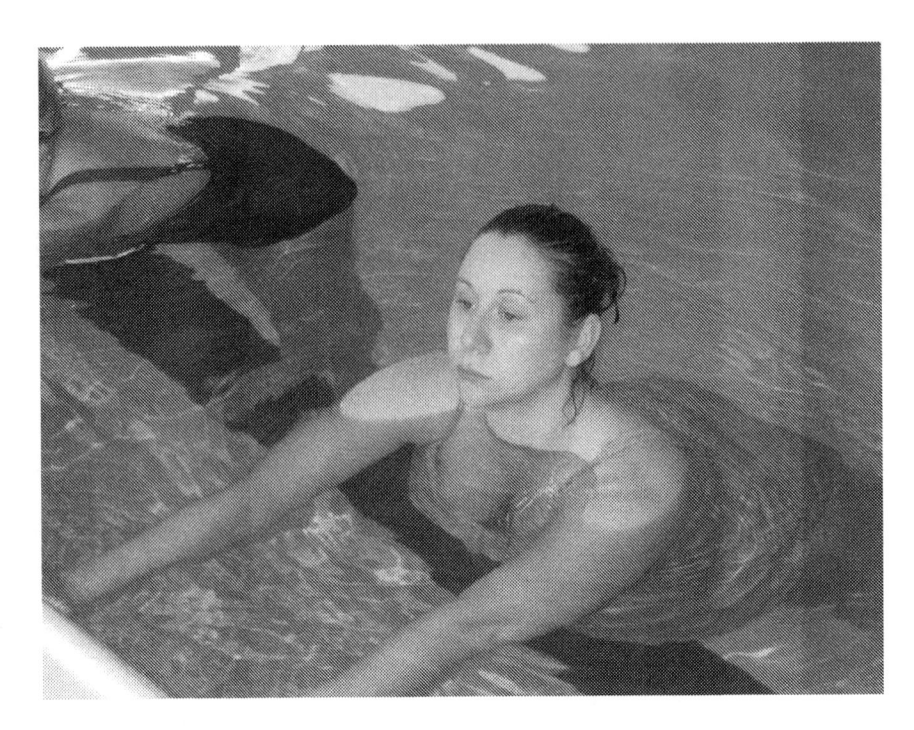

More shoulder work in Plank Pose
N.B. Student on left needs to step back to bring hips forward.

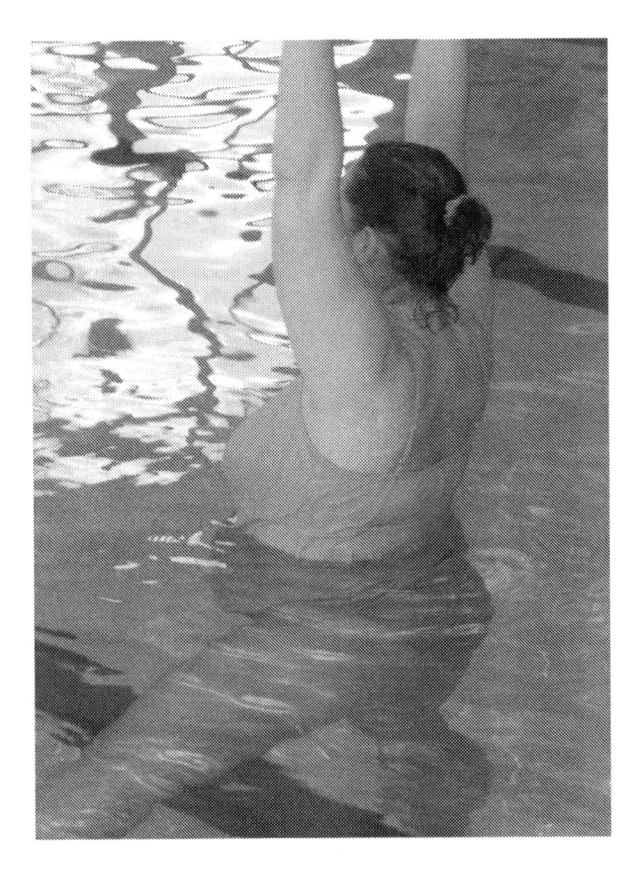

Tree pose for Composure and Balance

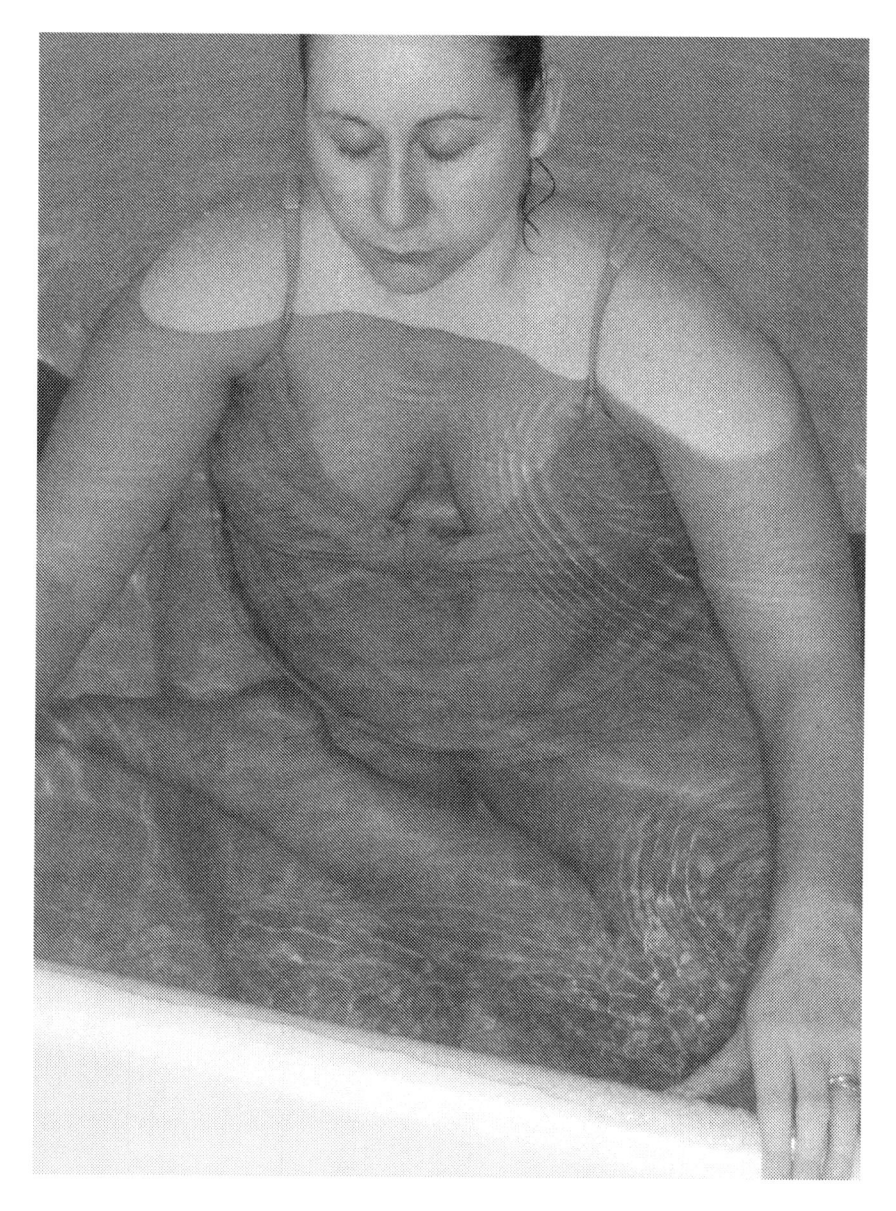

Sink into the hips and focus on the breath

"LIVING CREATURES ARE NOURISHED BY FOOD, AND FOOD IS NOURISHED BY RAIN; RAIN ITSELF IS THE WATER OF LIFE WHICH COMES FROM SELFLESS WORSHIP AND SERVICE"

BHAGAVAD GITA

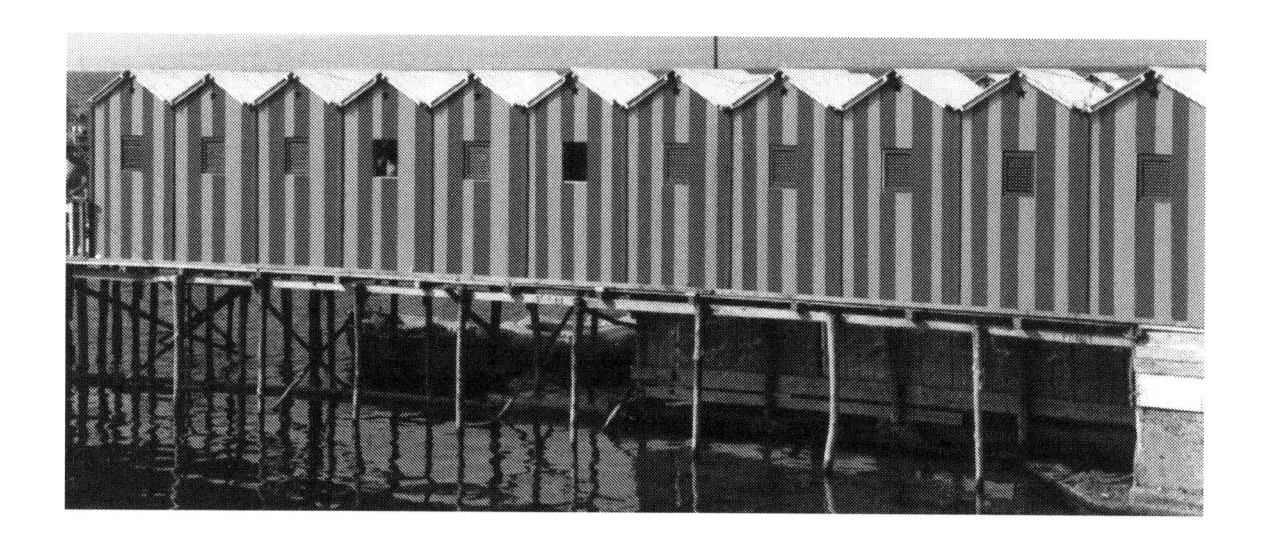

Aqua Yoga whilst on Vacation

    Very often this is a great place to start a yoga practice in the water. Life gets busy in the everyday working life, and trying something new whilst away from home may be the only chance people get. It is a great way for example for the 'stressed out executive', to unwind from the hectic pace of corporate life. It is a way for them to consciously slow down both physically and mentally and do something positive to bring balance back into their lives. It may be the only time that people can spare the time to check how they breathe and where the bias of the body actually is. Organized classes by hotels, and communities can be a great way to introduce this healthy activity into the pool.

    Choosing the right time to practice if there are not scheduled classes can pose a question, but should not pose a problem. There are usually some 'quiet times' in the pool where splashing and noise making is prohibited, if not, then ask for a quiet time which everyone can benefit from. The shallow wading pools may be available where you may be staying, and I like these to practice the monkey splits known as Hanuman stretch, and the more difficult arm balances.

    When I take the boys to Calistoga, practice is done in the lovely warm mineral pools, where I have the added benefit of the minerals clearing up my patch of eczema.

    Common sense should dictate not to practice in the midday sun if it is terribly hot, or without proper coverage with hat and sunglasses. Children can be encouraged to join in, and this may be a wonderful opportunity to introduce them to yoga, which is both educational and fun. The older children can help lead the younger ones, which can leave the parents more time to relax themselves, without having to listen to the dreaded 'Marco Polo' game for hours on end.

    As we get older, we become very rigid in our thinking process, and trying a new kind of activity that focuses so much on the way we breathe can help us develop a more carefree, childlike quality that makes us much nicer to be around. Lots of ladies in particular don't like the idea of getting their hair, or face wet, and so don't like to try floating, but they can float on an air bed if this is the case. My mother does not like to float by herself and so my father is very attentive in helping her to float in the pool. It is a very special time for them both, and a loving public display of their deep affection for one another that is not always shown on land. The surrender during floating is not only physical, but mental too, as people can release their intense thoughts that dominate their mind.

Sculling

The Torpedo scull that is practiced in synchronized swimming is a great asana for the experienced swimmer to experience "Uddiyana Bandha", or the lengthening of the inner body. Simply float on your back with upper arms close to the sides of the body and digits close together, drawing tiny figures of eight in the water. The leg muscles are engaged and pressed together and the hips lifted to the surface of the water. Arch the back as you sweep the arms overhead, and cultivate and sustain inner body length by drawing the belly and abdomen in and up. Then, open the fingers and point them downwards, waving from the wrists to propel yourself feet first. Keep the rib cage open, and the work in the legs, and don't forget to breathe.

You can become aware of the breath moving in the back of the body by sculling feet first with the tummy down, in reverse torpedo. It is more muscular, but helps to strengthen the upper body and open up the back. The elbows start off being close to the body, and then, in a scooping and pushing motion, rather like a squid, the body moves heel first across the pool. The legs need to be strong once again, and the heart lifted. Once you get going, try to lengthen from the back of the heart to the base of the scull.

Kids fun in the pool with Oyster

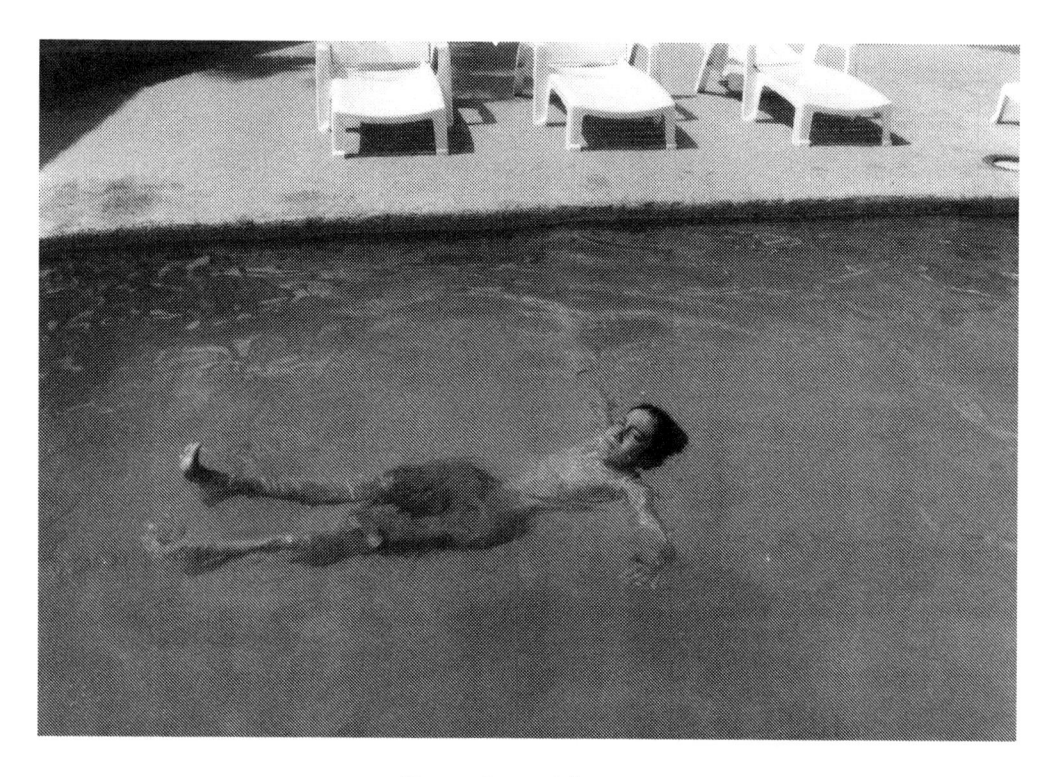

One minuet it's open.

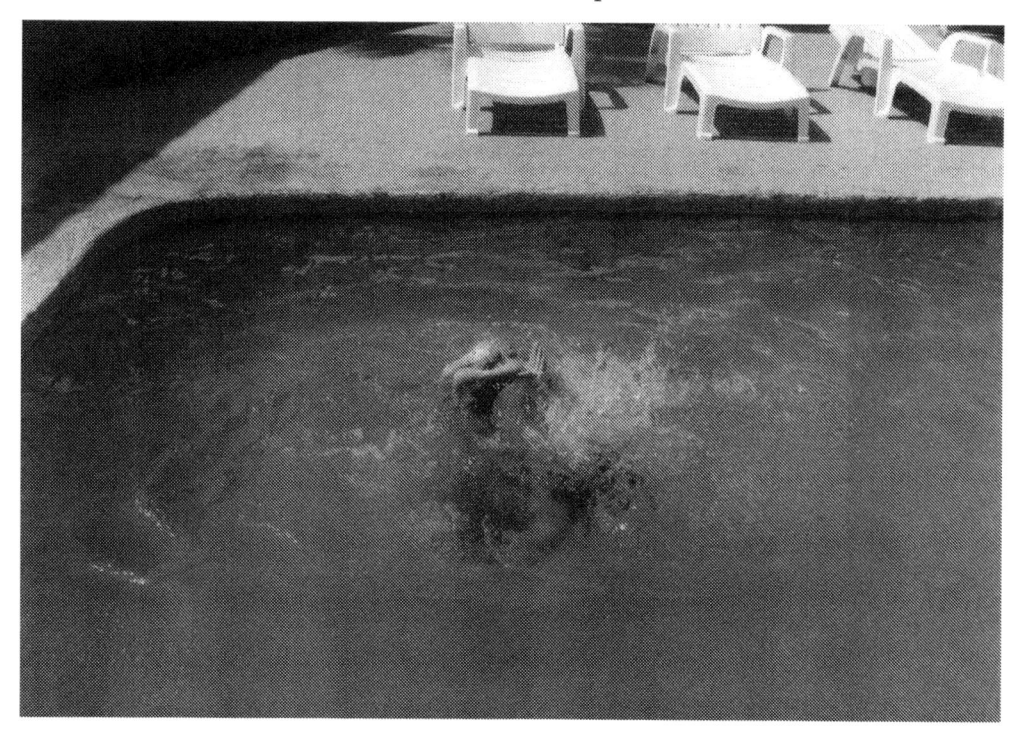

and the next it's closed. (extend arms out to sides and reach up.
On an inhale to touch toes as you sink down)

Older kids can help teach the younger ones about coordinating the breath and body.

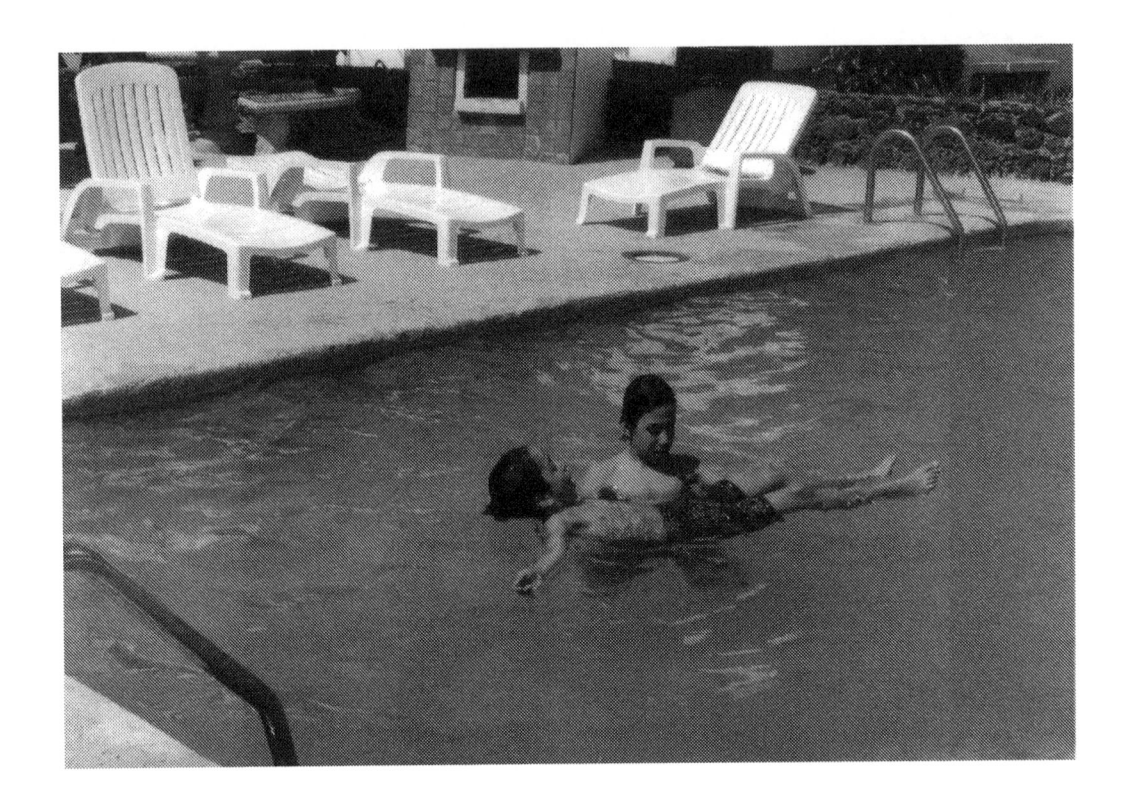

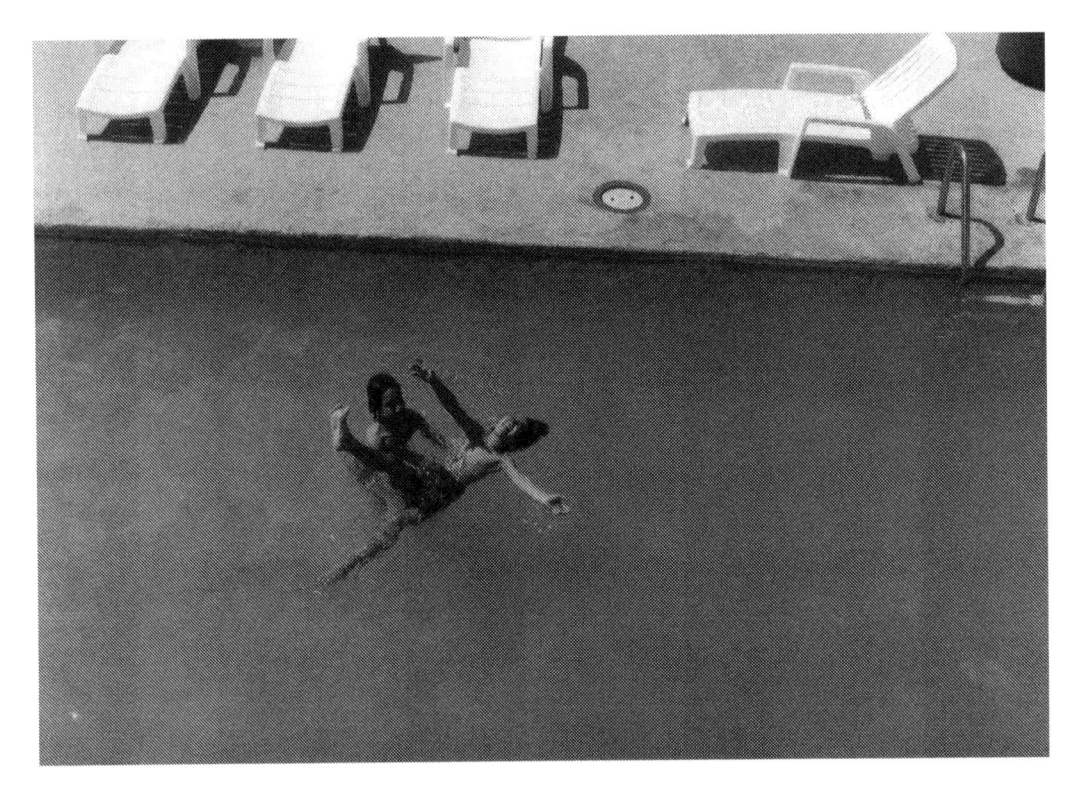

Handstand for the fearless kids helps them to strengthen their lungs.

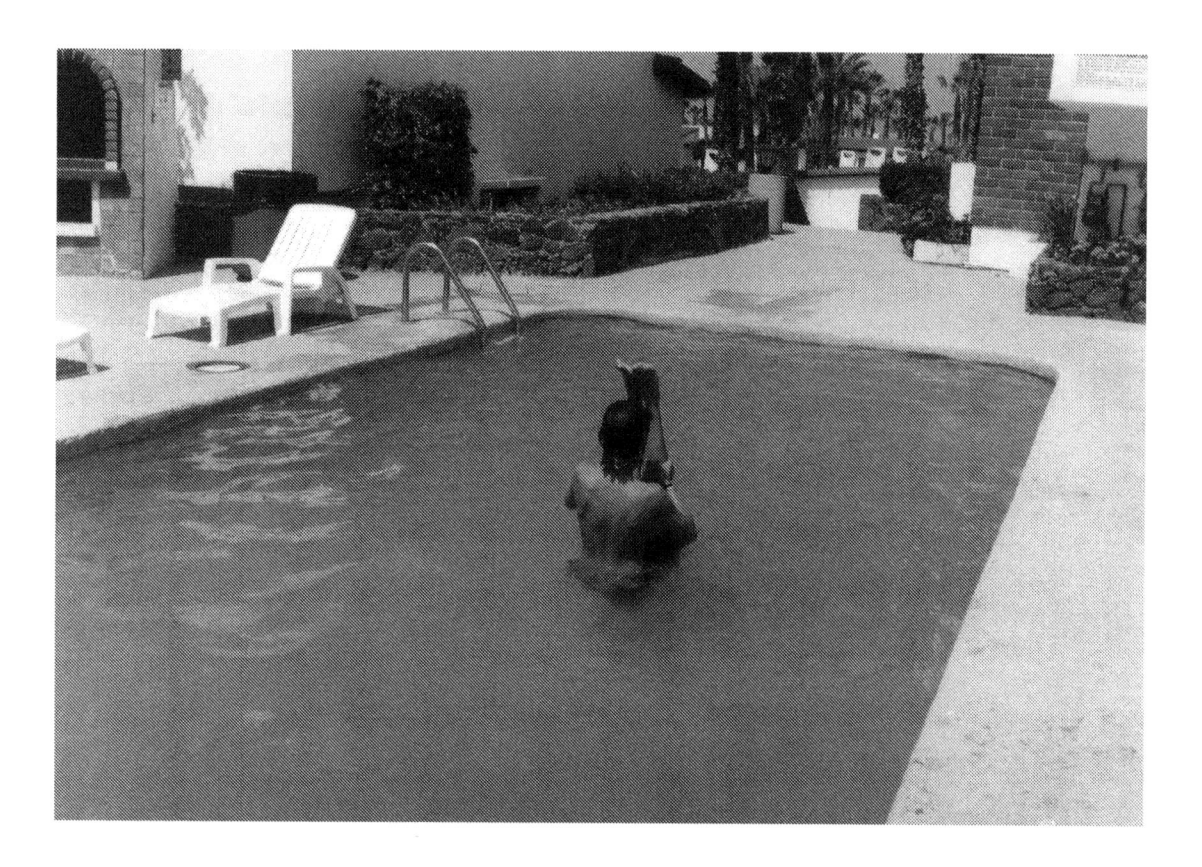

Fingers point towards toes and elbows press into loins.

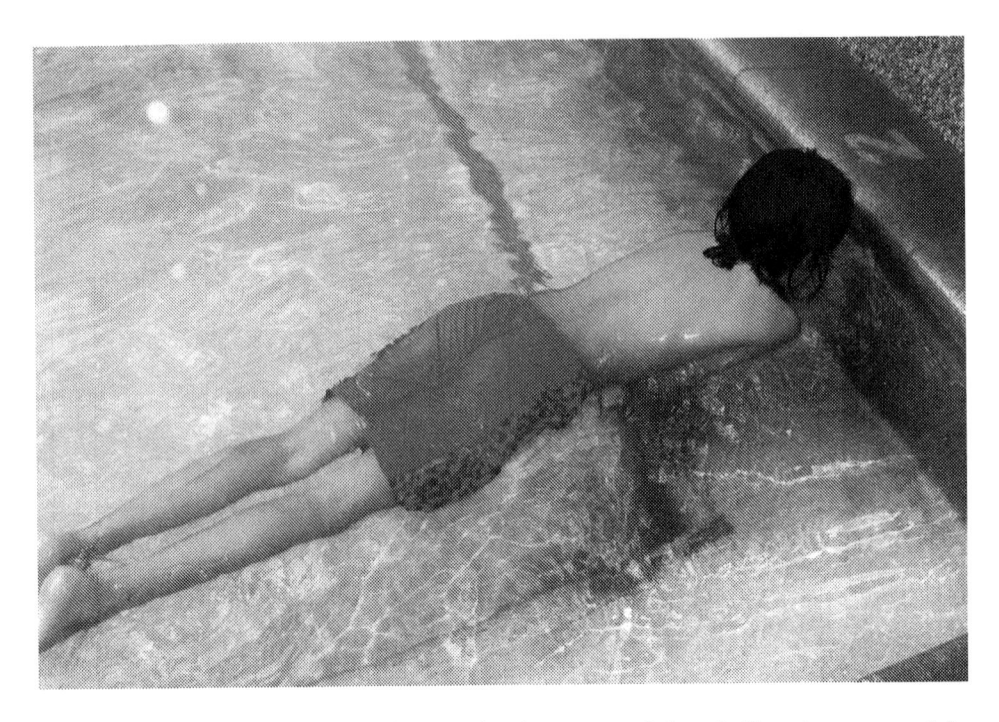

Using the steps can educate the student in the direction of this challenging pose – Mayurasana, which is one of the few asanas listed in the ancient Hatha Yoga Pradipika and Gherandha Samhita. It is said to help overcome many imbalances within the constitution.

"That was amazing, really amazing. The water tickled my forehead".

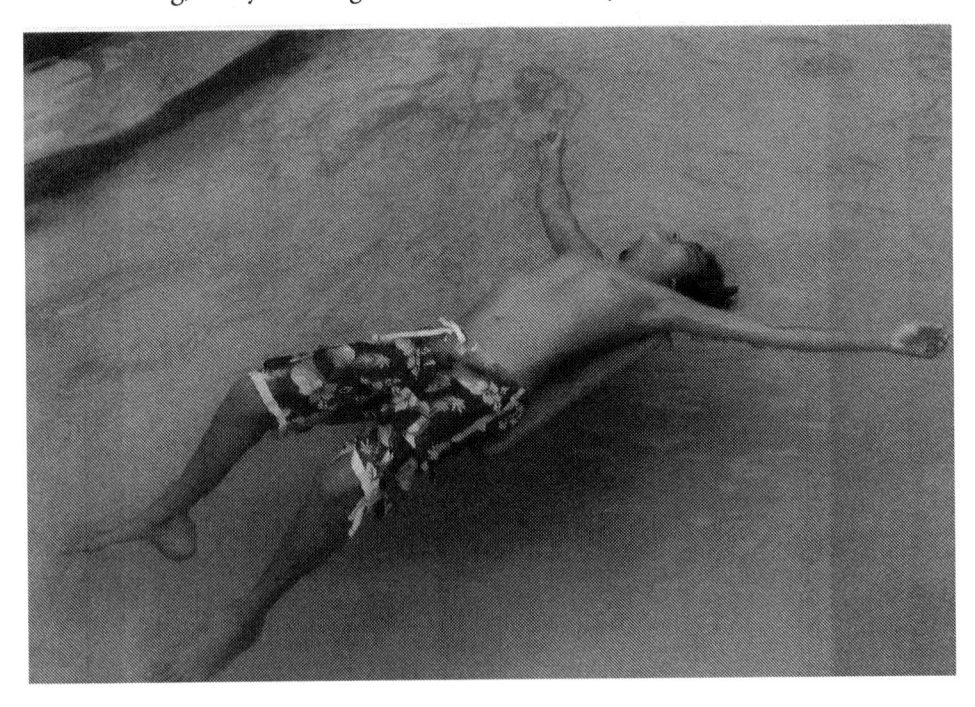

Savasana, or Corpse pose is another such ancient asana that is said to have enormous restorative attributes.

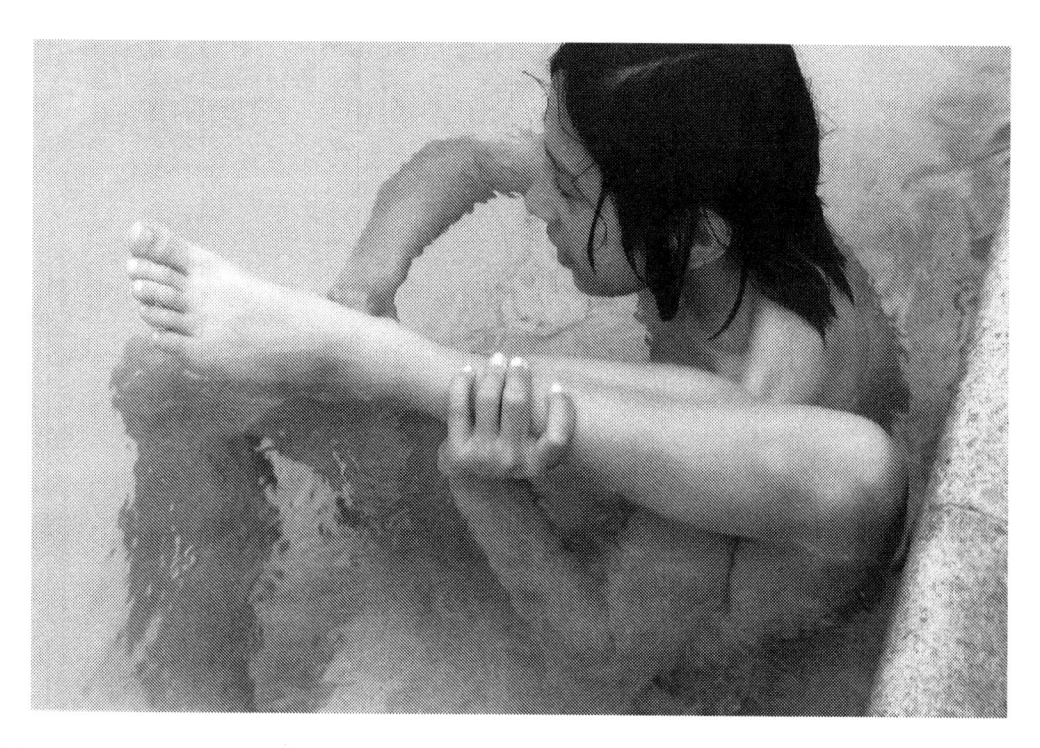

Children should be encouraged to work the hips open. Hip replacements are terribly common in the "western" body.

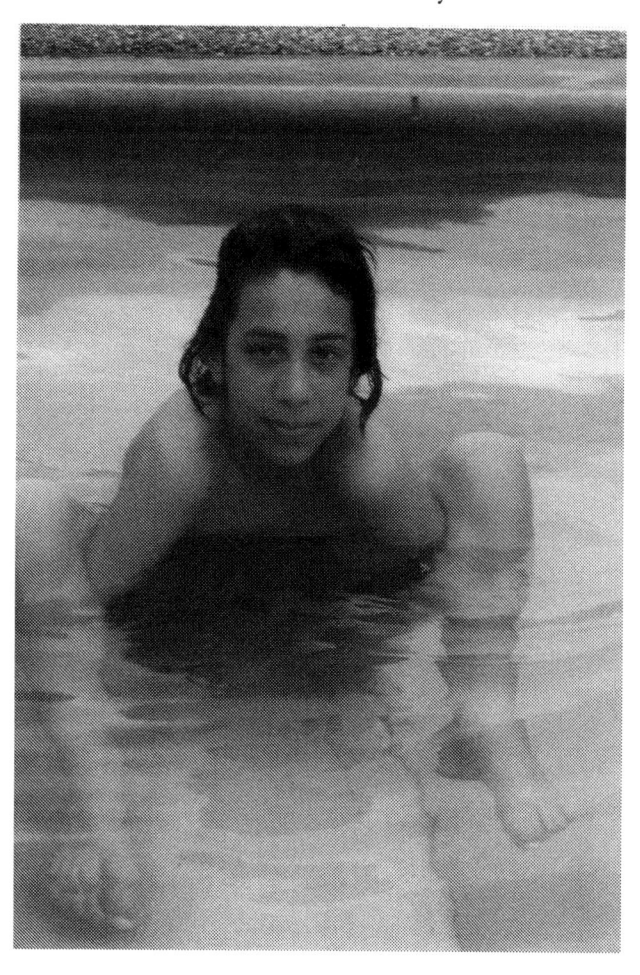

"YOU DON'T DROWN BY FALLING IN THE WATER; YOU DROWN BY STAYING THERE".

EDWIN LOUIS COLE

Aqua Yoga in the Hot Tub

The warm, soothing, swirling waters of a hot tub, can ease a tired and aching body. It's a nice place to unwind, gently stretch, or even to meditate for a short period. When I owned a house, I loved moon bathing and star gazing from the warm tub. What you can accomplish in the hot tub, like anywhere else, is subject to where you are at mentally, emotionally and physically. The dimensions and accessibility of the tub itself is also a factor, as is the temperature, (on what is I hope an obvious note, the head should not be placed under the water in a hot tub). It can be a great place to reflect on life generally.

Here are a few just a few suggestions for working in the tub. Opening the hips and shoulders, along with extension of the spine can be some areas that can be worked here especially well. Do make sure that you hydrate properly though. My son told me that at the full moon, when we know people are crazier than normal, people pee less, and this causes pressure in the brain. Whether that is true or not, we need to hydrate more as a general rule, and then even more if we use a hot tub.

Arnold L.Lieber M.D., in his book, 'The Lunar Effect', talks about the human body and how it is affected by the ebb and flow of the gravitational and electromagnetic tides, in exactly the same way that the earth is. There is said to be a greater tendency to bleed more at full or new moons when we are injured. Just like the movements in the ocean, gravity has an effect upon the water mass in the body.

If we reflect or tarka, listing our emotions and reactions following the cycles of the moon, we can make great advances in understanding the imbalance within us. Any female who has her period around a full moon can relate to the misery of a bloated feeling. Tempers often ignite in the seemingly sweetest of people. Expectant mothers too can be volatile emotionally which corresponds to their increase in body fluids. The same gravitational pull ensures that men are not exempt from the lunar effects, only in some cases they hide it a little better.

Some suggestions

* Moon bathe at the full moon and reflect upon the day's events, or the events of the last lunar cycle from the new moon. How have you reacted to other people's thoughts, words, and actions? How could you have changed the way you thought, spoke or acted? Keeping a journal of these reflections can reveal a great deal about our personality, and what triggers emotionality.

* Practice mantra (thought form), and especially EEEE mantra with the jets gently pounding the back. Mantra allows us to feel the vibration of the mantra in the head and throat, and has a balancing, calming effect, that induces serenity. Simply inhale through the nostrils and exhale chanting EEEE audibly for as long as it remains strong and clear. Then stop abruptly, before the sound fizzles out. The sound should be of equal intensity from start to finish. Then, just concentrate at the sun center between the eyebrows and let the breath breathe you effortlessly. It is a nice purifying practice for the subtle body as it shakes negative thought forms from the aura, and even strengthens it, making us less reactive to other people and their energy.

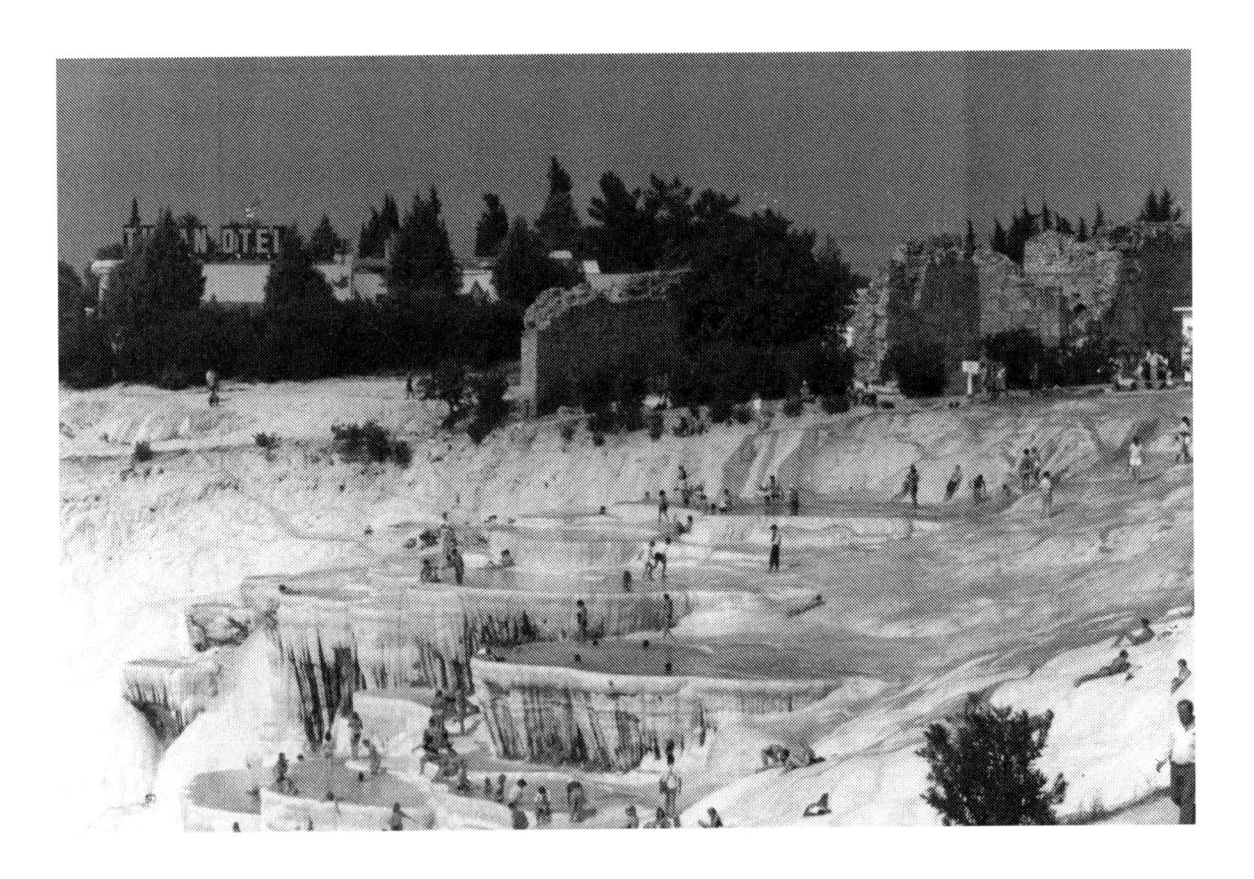

Hot tub

Gentle stretching can be done here

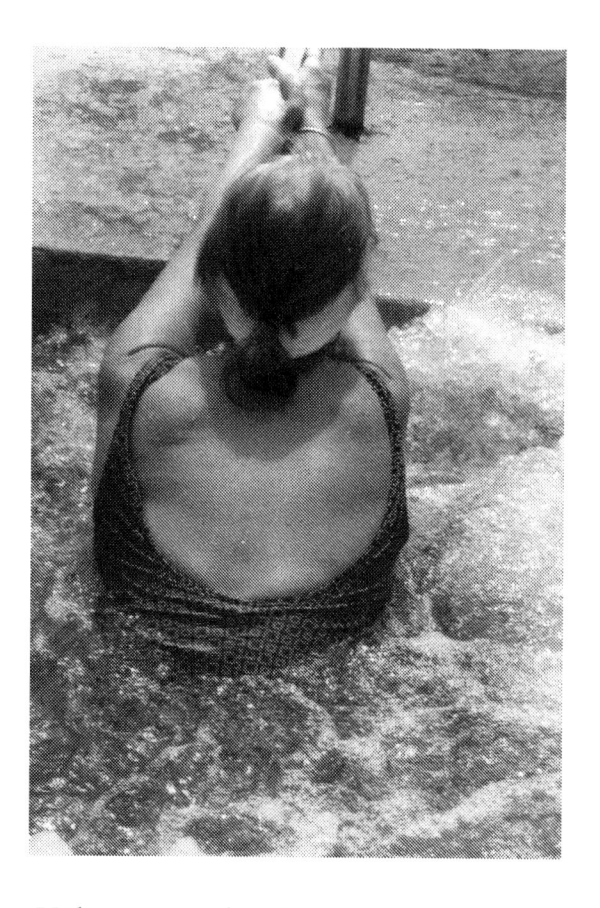

Utilize steps and seating areas as appropriate

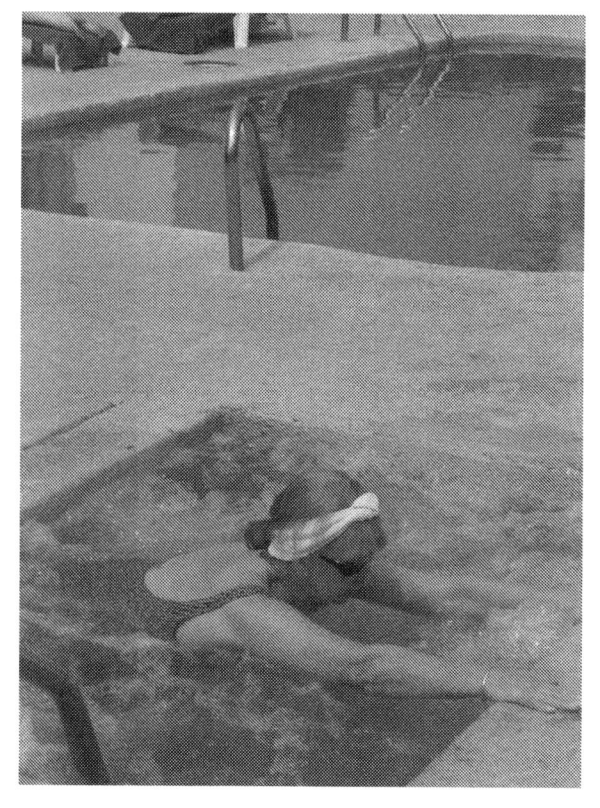

The bubbles from jets can add an extra inner massage and tone the skin.

Reflection as you relax

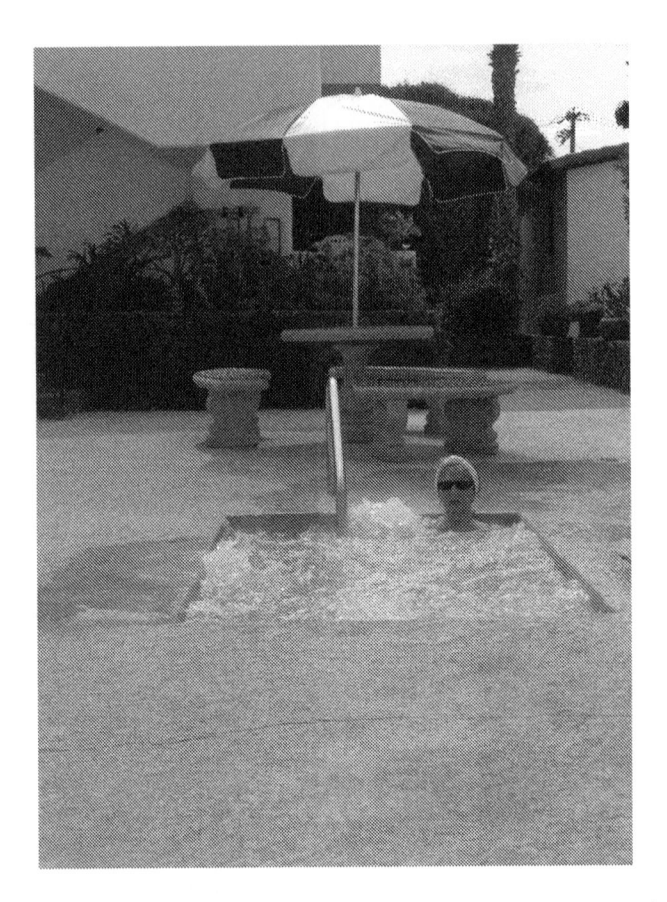

Watch the habits your child is forming in his posture and help them change it by becoming more aware. This is a gift for them for the rest of their life. Learning to breath right and stand and sit correctly.

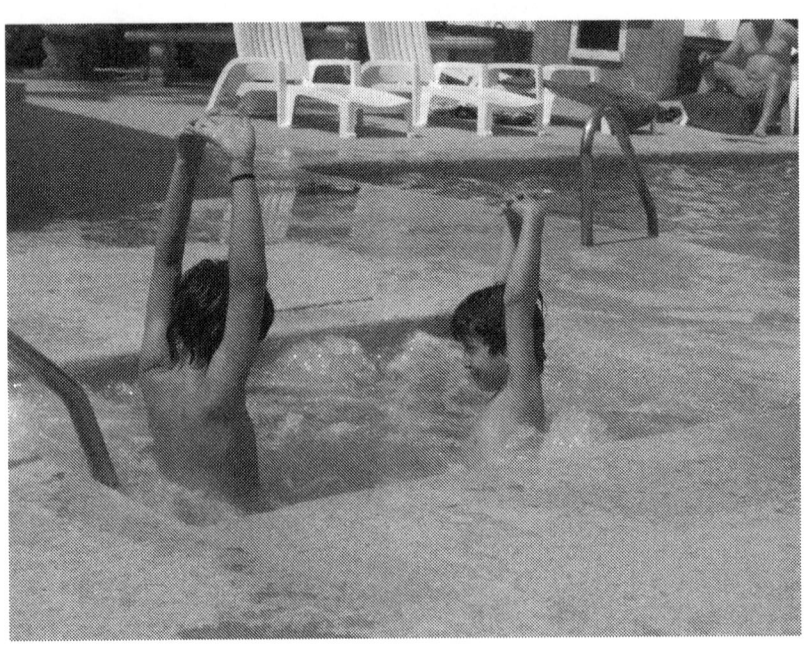

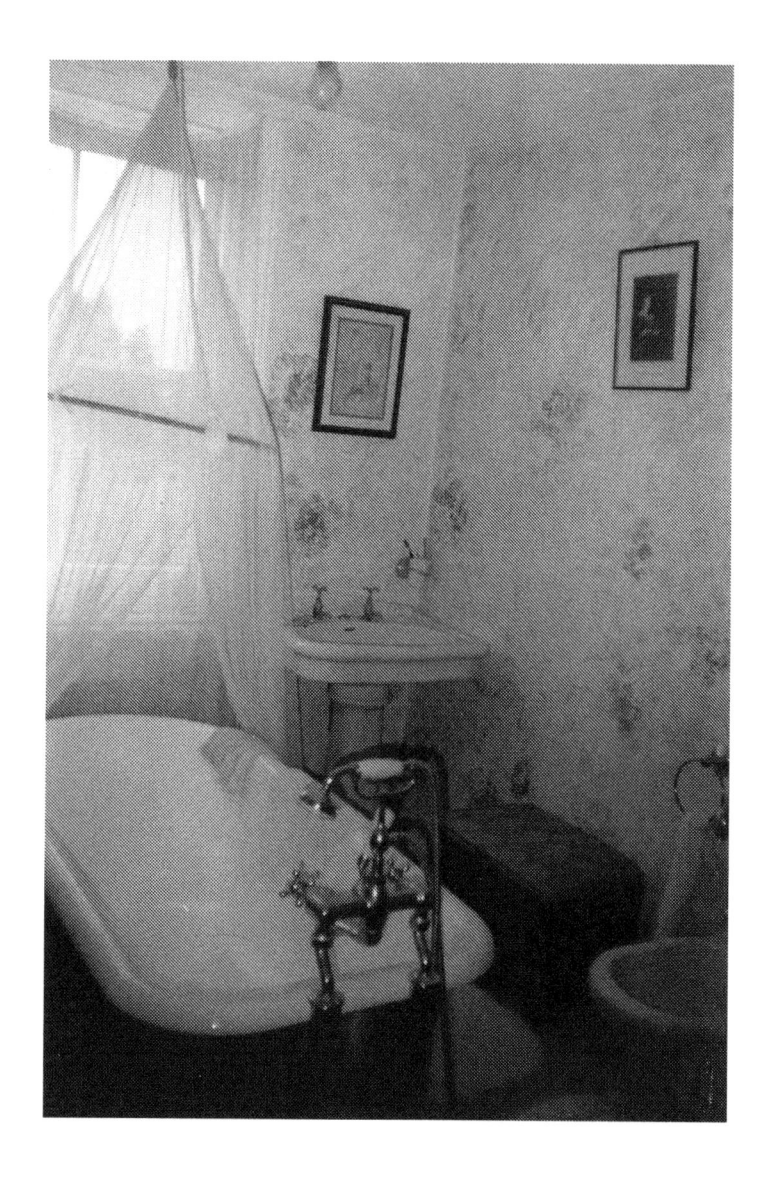

Saucha or Purity of mind and body is something we need to cultivate. For a bathroom to become a sanctuary and place of rejuvenation it should be clean, free from dampness and odors, and not be cluttered with dirty linens.

"IF YOU WOULD SWIM ON THE BOSOM OF THE OCEAN OF TRUTH, YOU MUST REDUCE YOURSELF TO A ZERO"

GANDHI

Kriya Yoga in the Bathroom

Kriya yoga is all about cultivating conscious actions, and the mystic would even consider showering and bathing a conscious ritual that can help yoke the mind and body. My Paramguru recommends showering and changing out of work clothes as soon as you get home. This is because we pick up other people's subtle karmic particles when we are in their company. Most people don't unfortunately love their work, so showering is an important ritual to perform in order not to subject the spouse, or other family members to the negative energy collected during the day. The ritual is simple. Simply allow the water to run over the crown of the head to the feet, and visualize the negative energy being washed away. The same work clothes should not be put on, as they carry the vibrations like a dog carries fleas.

Locking the bathroom door may provide the only sanctuary in a busy household, and time spent languishing in a warm bubbly bath can be precious. Often life seems much better after a good soak, because the emotionality has lost its destructive force, especially if Epsom salts are added to the bath water. The eyes are associated with the fire element and water conducts the heat of the fire. Kriyanandaji recommends flicking water on the face to abate the thoughts that keep churning in the mind. Even if you don't have time to shower or bathe, just washing the face and hands can make you feel better. The hand contact charges the water, which soothes the eyes and optic nerves, which are connected to the brain. Eye baths occasionally with a drop of rosewater can refresh eyes. Details can be obtained from good local health stores these days. Washing the feet regularly during the day is said to increase vitality and contentment, and washing before bedtime especially can help aid sound sleep.

Turkish baths have been in Europe since about the 1850's, and there are still some that can be found, for example Bath in England, where some have been restored. The word Hammam means bathroom, and these are communal baths, typically not co-ed. In Ayurveda, which is a sacred science of self-healing closely related to yoga, there are many healing rituals that are available to improve health and well being. In the process of Pancha Karma, one would undergo steam therapy (svedana) and enema's as a part of a spring or summer detox program.
On a daily basis, we can use the neti pot, which are easily obtained at health stores and have had a wonderful effect on many of my students. It involves passing salt water from one nostril to the other and is regarded as the cleansing process within the forehead. A spot of sesame oil can be applied after the treatment. The instructions come with the pot and are simple to follow. If you swim in the sea the likely hood is that you will clear the nasal passages by default almost, but try thinking about it being a conscious kriya or action to intensify the benefits on a subtle level.

Many people, especially men, like to read on the toilet and this is not a good habit. Newspapers are considered the worst things to read as when you read, you lock yourself into any negative emotions that are no longer current. Holding on to the past in the same way that you are holding on to the stool that is toxic. Reading brings the energy to the head rather than where it is needed, and it tends to encourge people to stay on the toilet longer than is necessary. Washing the anus is thought to be more effective than just using paper alone, which can irritate the skin. As the water is an electrical conductor, it draws the energy to the surface, and allows it to be distributed and stimulate the nervous system, including the brain. The nerves of the digestive tract connect to the plexus in the anus. Traditionally the yogi would use the toilet before meditation. A constitution that has problems passing waste is a big blind spot in one's practice. Withholding pee causes unnecessary pain to the bladder, aching genitals, headaches, bloatedness and diseases of the genito-urinary system. Delayed defecation causes more of the same type of problems along with additional anger. In Europe, it is common to have a bidet in the bathroom but in America they are not so common. Space can be an issue. You can however buy a shower head attachment that can be fitted to the toilet system so that the anus can be washed. My father picked one up at a local Persian store and installed it for about thirty dollars.

Steam showers are a wonderful way to bring the spa environment into your own home. I like to add a few drops of eucalyptus or a bunch of fresh leaves to the shower, especially at the onset of a cold. In the Middle East, the Turkish Hammam is part of everyday life. There are usually a series of rooms that people gather in, moving deeper to its center in progressively hotter rooms. There is a relaxing warm room where ladies can remove unwanted hair, apply henna and face packs etc.. Then they proceed into a hotter room and may take turns scrubbing one another with a mitt to remove dead skin cells. They use buckets of warm and cold water to slosh over themselves, and continue moving freely about the rooms sometimes for hours talking, relaxing and contemplating life. If you are going as a tourist, avoid the so called, Hammam's in Hotels. These are geared towards the naive foreigners, and do not do justice to the experience of the sacred ritual of bathing that dates back to the Roman times. In the Roman Empire there were thought to be about one thousand public baths and pools.

Salt rubs are inexpensive and help to exfoliate the largest organ of the body, namely the skin. Adding a few drops of your favorite essential oil to the running bath water will fill the whole room with scent quickly, and so start its work all the sooner. Good quality pure oils can be found in all good health stores. Apart from trusty lavender oil which is usually with me in my bag at all times, clary sage I have found to be extremely beneficial in the bath to ease menstrual pain. Also that, with a carrier oil such as almond rubbed onto the tummy and a hot water bottle, can ease the discomfort considerably.

In Europe many of the hospitals now offer birthing pools for the expectant mum. If they don't have them, they are very easy to rent and well worth the bother of self- assembly.

Saucha or purity is one of the things in yoga we try to cultivate. The element of water is linked to the svadisthana, or Jupiter chakra at the sacrum and is associated with expansion.

We can reap superb results in terms of harmony and contentment by embodying the teachings of yoga, and bringing them into every facet of our lives. Actually, we can strive to be fully conscious and aware in each and every breath.

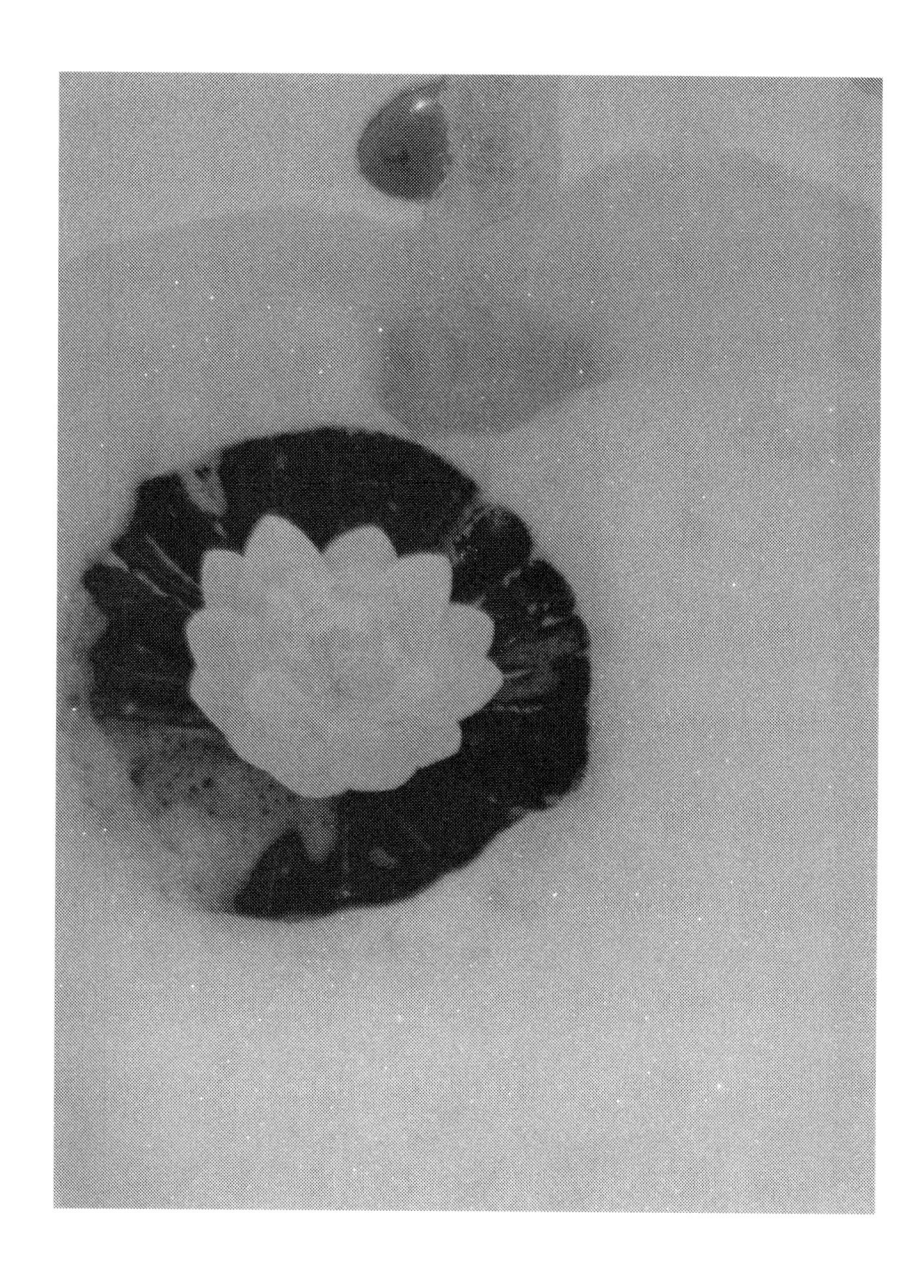

The bathroom may be the only chance you have of being alone and quiet. Enjoy this time and relax and renew in the purifying waters.

Patanjali's 8 limbs of Self Transformation

(An ancient text that outlines the yoga discipline)

The Yoga Sutra's of Patanjali are short sayings, contained within four small books, that help the practitioner understand the steps on the path of Self-Revelation. They were compiled around 200 A.D., and are the key teachings that the student who wants to understand more than just the physical postures (often called yoga), would study.

Within the books, the very foundations of the practice are explained, and are known as the '8 limbs'. The first lists that which we should try to control in our lives, and the second, that which we need to develop more of in our lives. They are called the Yamas and Niyamas. We should have some degree of a sane lifestyle that is conducive to understanding, and this is what the practice of the Yamas and Niyamas brings about. A desire to live in accord with others, is as important as becoming more familiar with the physical body and how it breathes. In other words, the system or 8 limbs are not to be practiced sequentially, but simultaneously. The whole system is known as Yoga, and Hatha is two parts of that system. The two components of Hatha, being postures and breath/prana yama (control).

Outer practices

1. Restraints (yamas) Non-Violence, Non-Stealing, Control of vital Energies, Non-Greed, Non-Lying.

2. Observances (niyamas) Purity, Contentment, Self-discipline, Self-Study, Attunement to inner-Self.

3. Asanas/Postures

4. Pranayama/ Control of life energies known as Prana, through breath work.

Inner Practices

5. Sense Withdrawal

6. Concentration

7. Meditation

8. Samadhi (some call it super-consciousness, and many other translations but by Paramguru prefers to call it Samadhi).

The 8 limbs, or disciplines of yoga, can still be explored by the ardent student in the water environment, if they have some degree of Self- awareness.

The only difference between any two students is the length of time it takes them on their spiritual path, and what they experience along the way. We should not limit our thinking to where one's physical practice is. Attitude is everything. What may be appropriate and enjoyable for one soul may not be so for another.

Any student will absorb some of what they see the teacher has embodied. It will be a transmission of consciousness whether they are aware of it or not. Every person affects us in some way. Like a chakra or energy center, they either cause our consciousness to expand, or contract. The very small percentage of free will that most humans use, gives us the freedom to react or respond. The problem is, most of us do not recognize this, because of our vested self- interest and emotionality, and get caught up in a cyclical patterning of cause and effect, known as karma. If we drive recklessly all the time, at some point it will have an effect. Perchance an accident or a ticket. Karma is not the law of retribution.

The postures and the control of prana, or life energies, link together in a sacred dance of the breath on land and in the water, and can help remove the negativity we may have, (contract and dissolve the thoughts) or expand our mind to be able to think a new thought and solve the problem in our life. (expansion of new thoughts)   A problem is only something that we have yet to solve.

Many people have no enthusiasm for life, and are confined into the more
dense lower chakras, that can emanate fearful, limited thoughts at Muladhara
or Saturn chakra at the tail bone,
Jealousy and greedy thoughts at Svadisthana or Jupiter chakra at the base of
the spine,or
Desire and anger filled thoughts at Manipura or Mars chakra at the navel
area.

As we become more content we can experience the positive effects of the more subtle etheric chakras that are located at the heart (Venus) and throat (mercury), as well as balancing the lower chakras. We will become more loving, compassionate and commune with others much better.

Inner and outer contentment is a lifestyle and attitude that stems from us being comfortable with our human body and mind. Excepting the limitations of both, but recognizing that a new thought will move us away from who and what other people, or our own minds have told us we are. (keep telling a child they are naughty for example, and they will oblige, and also only think of themselves as being naughty. The danger here is that they will perpetuate the insanity, and probably teach their children the same.)   How often do we think we sound like our mother or father?

If we start to view ourselves more positively, we can project that out to other people. We move away from our self invested ego to something greater than ourselves, which is Life.

The inner limbs of yoga can of course be experienced in, or near water. They are Sense Withdrawal, Concentration, Meditation and Samadhi. The experienced student can explore this for themselves. The novice should learn them first on land from a qualified instructor.

Kriya Yoga is a discipline and a discovery of our greater Self, in each and every breath we breathe.

The below average yoga student will perhaps not be interested in anything other that improving their body, and that is great if yoga gives them that, which it will, but the student that is showing an interest in understanding why they are feeling so positive and alive, may express an interest in learning more. It will probably not be appropriate to expand on asana and breath work for the majority of classes, but for select workshops it is possible.

Interested students can be encouraged to read books, or use a computer to do some studying for themselves. There are many teachers available in most areas where they can find like- minded souls and continue learning.

" WATER IS THE ONLY DRINK FOR A WISE MAN ".

HENRY DAVID THOREAU (1817 -1862)
American naturalist, poet and philosopher

" WHISKEY IS FOR DRINKING, WATER IS FOR FIGHTING OVER",

ATTRIBUTED TO MARK TWAIN

A small boy appreciates free, clean water not far from it's source

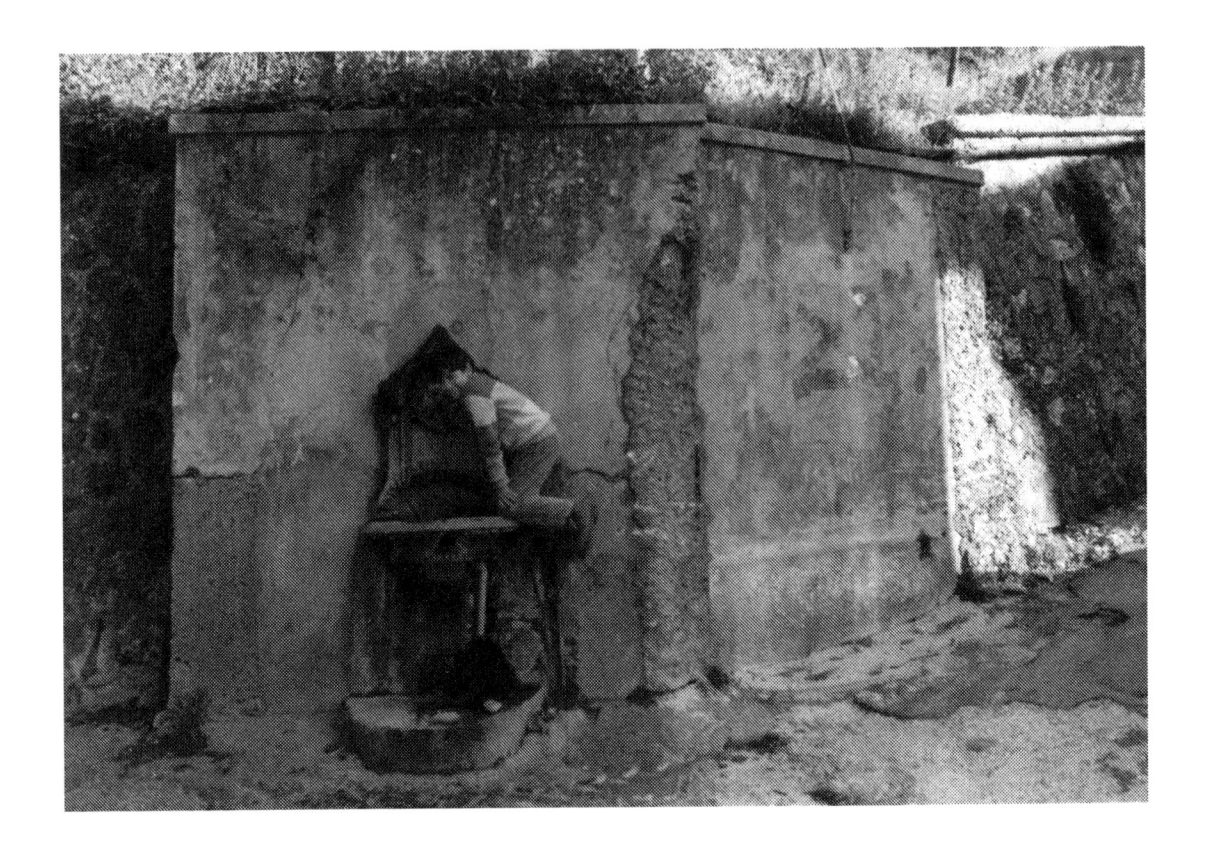

"A FOUNTAIN OF JOY
MUST GUSH OUT OF THE SOUL OF THY MIND
AND SPREAD SPRAYS OF FINE SMILES
RUNNING IN ALL DIRECTIONS".

From Yogananda's poem, "Fountain of Smiles - Whispers from Eternity."

The Water You Drink

Most of the tap water has some degree of contamination in it, and has been recycled many times, so is said to lack vital life force or Prana. This is one reason that yogis prefer to drink water from the purest source possible. Mountain spring water is well worth the extra money spent and is better than distilled, purified or filtered.

About 6-8 glasses should be drunk each day. More in hot weather, or if you are fasting. This keeps the body nice and moist, and helps with the process of elimination which is a vital process that eliminates toxins from the body, and prevents a build up of mucus and amma. The average person does not drink enough water, and it is needed to help regulate the body temperature as well as lubricate the joints. If you drink caffeine, more water needs to be drunk.

It is a good practice to take a glass of warm water first thing in the morning to help facilitate a bowel movement, (cold water cannot dissolve some particles) Lemon juice can be added to it if you prefer.

This allows the blood to flow more freely around the body and into the skin, the largest organ.

Most of us do not live near a clean water source unfortunately. I remember when I lived in Italy, close to a fountain that spewed ribbons of fresh mineral water, smelling of rotten eggs. The smell was horrid, yet it tasted so sweet and delicious. Locals would come every day and fill up their empty bottles. Once you have become a connoisseur of water, it is very unpleasant to go back to standard tap water. Be wary of the big companies that sell water that has no connection to its source. This seems to be the only type of water I have noticed, on sale at airports, in American gyms and health clubs. What a pity.

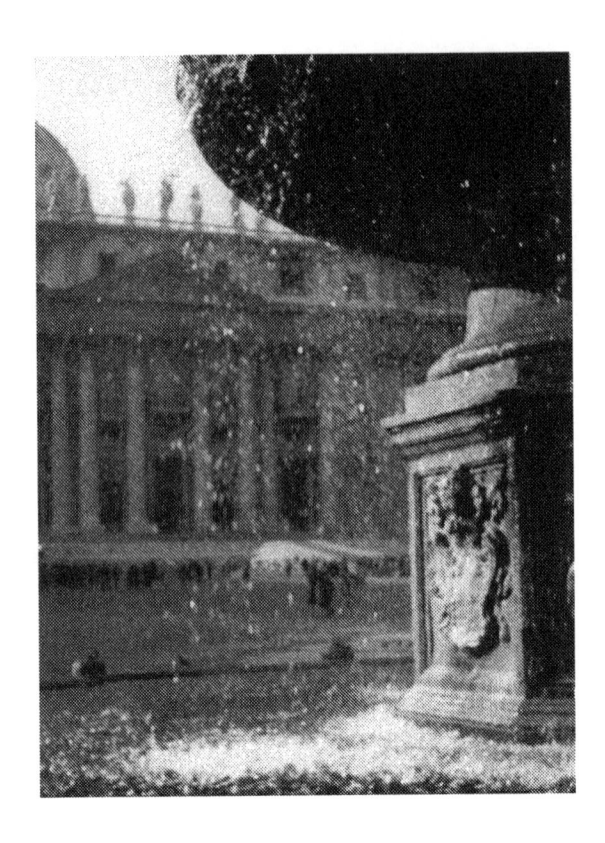

Sound Therapy

Fountains are a marvelous addition to any home and garden, and bring a relaxing element into the environment that is coveted by placement experts, in both the Indian and Chinese traditions.

We don't all live by the sea, yet the sound of the ocean is very popular for therapists and body workers, as it soothes their clients. Listening to the rain can also be very relaxing to some people, especially if you are warm and cozy inside. The smell of fresh earth after the rain stops, is like the smell of a new day dawning. Large waterfalls crashing down hundreds of feet, sounds like the sacred mantra OM manifesting from the subtle realms.

Small spaces can accommodate a water fountain or pond. The ideal place for a pond, according to Indian Vastu is in the north or north-eastern part of the garden. Vishnu, the element water and Jupiter are associated with this direction. If the water feature is above ground, the experts suggest a south-west aspect may be more auspicious. A flow of water from east to west or west to east will generate negative ions and freshen the air.

Vastu Shastra (dwelling science) is the ancient Indian science of harmonious living similar to Feng Shui. It is the art of design, placement and building that helps to direct the flow of energies into and around the home. As in the great yoga lineages, Vastu was originally transmitted orally from guru to disciple. One does not need to intellectualize about the effect of the science of placement, merely try it and experience the results for one's self.

The last house I lived in, when it was originally on the market, was terribly neglected and if it were not for it's potential and the fact that it had many well established plants in the garden with the orange blossom in bloom, I would have run a mile. Even after remodeling, there was a lot of heavy negative energy from the previous owners and the spirit of a woman in my kitchen that did not want to move on. The children and I did a simple house blessing that involves first cleaning the house, especially the floor, and rearranging a few things. Blessed water was sprinkled around the house, especially near the doors and closets which seemed to do the trick. Intention plays a key role here, and any family member that the ritual is useless should not be in the house whilst you perform the ritual, as they will tend to negate any positive effect. Any priest or spiritual worker would be glad to help you bless your home and make it a happier place to dwell. If you are doing the ritual yourself, you can bless the water that should be in a pretty vessel just for that occasion, by reciting a prayer or mantra that is meaningful to you.

In the garden, a trench filled with water will indicate if positive energy is in the land if a flower head spins clockwise in it. A counter clockwise direction is not considered auspicious in the northern hemisphere. The opposite is true in the southern. (water as it drains away down the plug hole, has the same directional flow in the earth's hemisphere's)

In the house, the ideal plan would include a kitchen in the south-east direction and a bathroom and toilet in the north west or east.

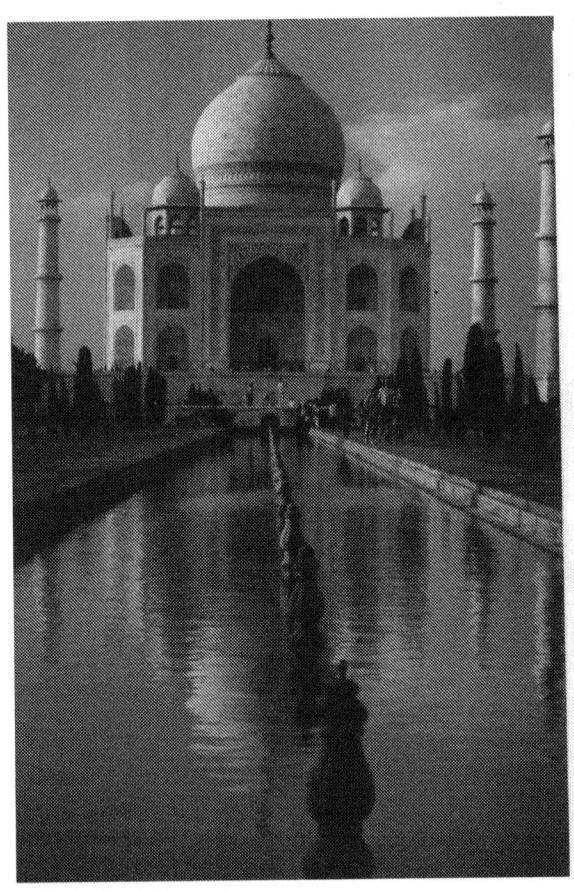

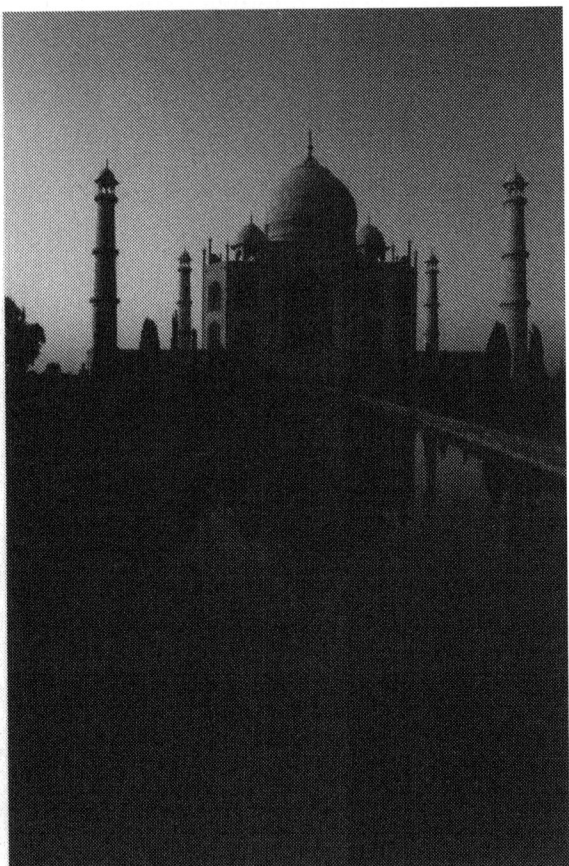

The Taj Mahal

    Although a Muslim design, rather than Hindu, it's design and how it fits in with the Vastu Shasta rules makes it an incredible place of reflection and meditation. It honors man's architectural genius, and actually enhances nature's beauty as it unites with it. The Taj takes on many colors and moods during the course of a day and is reflected in the large pool.

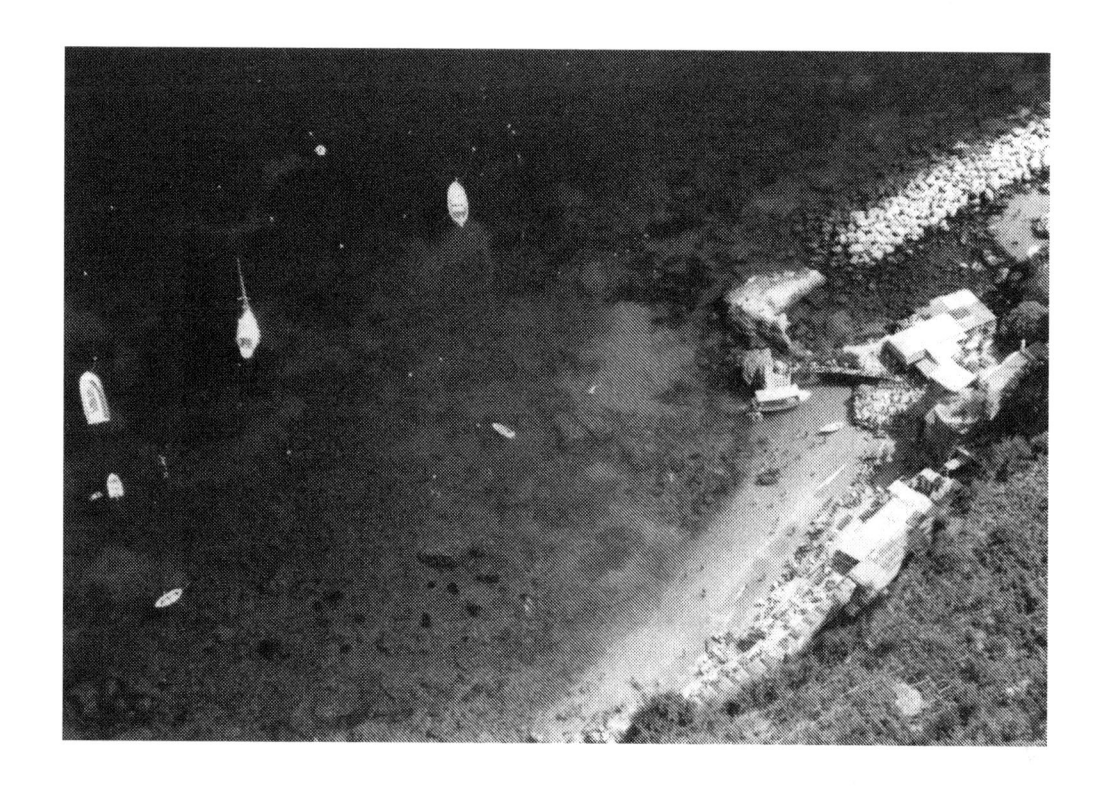

Snorkeling is great for listening to breathing patterning.

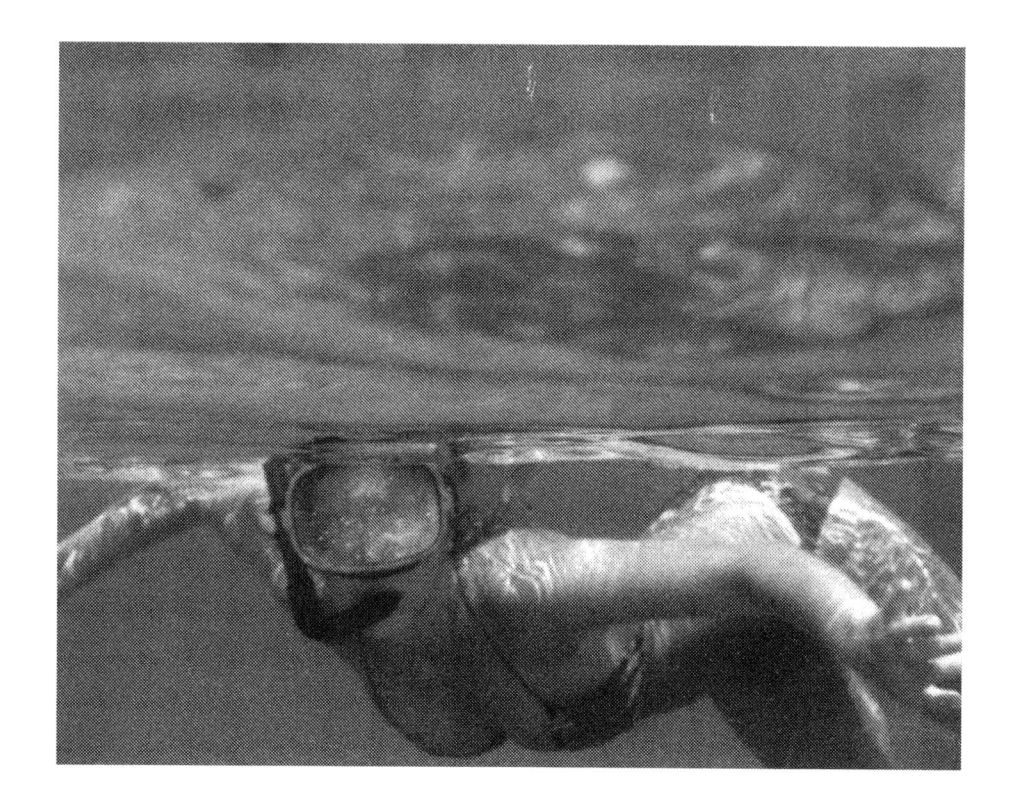

Pranayama (life force control)

Snorkeling in the water gives us an excellent opportunity to hear the aspirated sound of ujjayi pranayama, known as victorious breath. This is the type of breath that should be heard internally in our hatha yoga practice rather than externally.
The sound of thundering silence in the ears, is very similar to that heard when one closes off the ears in yoni mudra. (A sense withdrawal technique)

Sound waves travel a great distance in the water. Poor whales know this very well as some of them get disorientated, by careless testing of bombs many thousands of miles away. Thought forms travel in much the same way as sound waves. No defined boundaries of space and time, so we need to be more mindful of the thoughts we think. Our awareness of how we are breathing, and the unconscious shortening of the inhale or exhale, should be examined and corrected if possible, through breathing techniques. There are many books available that cover this subject very well. Once we become more aware of our inner universe, we hear different sounds. Perceiving firstly, the sound of the ocean. The process of breath control is an involution. It helps to balance the body and mind as we absorb more oxygen and prana. The process allows us to turn around in consciousness and become more aware of our inner, subjective universe. If you like swimming underwater, it is a lovely way to connect with other life forms, especially if you are in warm, clear water.

The key benefits of practicing breathing techniques is that the body becomes more nourished and vitalized, especially the circulatory and nervous systems.

In an Aqua Yoga class, or any yoga class, the student that is not breathing correctly will tend to become frustrated very easily. This is usually a reflection of lifestyle. To the degree we are ranting and raving in our daily lives, is the degree that we will have difficulty controlling the breathing patterning. Through practice and controlled breathing patterns however, the every day breath can be changed, and there too our level of serenity.

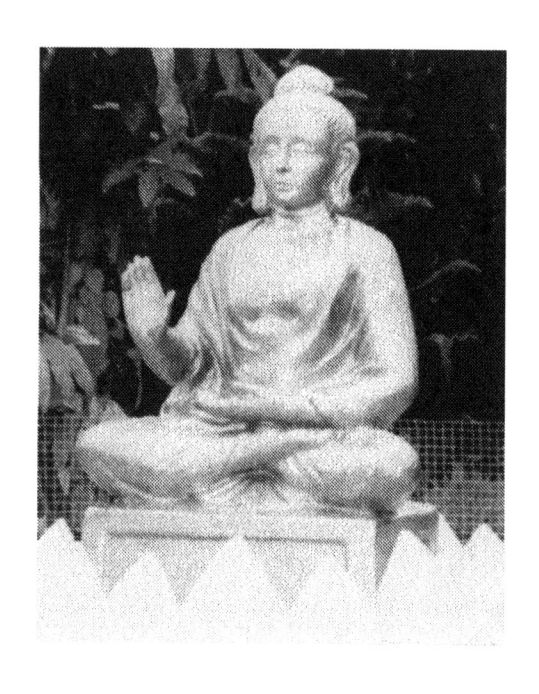

"WHEN THE BREATH FINALLY REACHES THE TOP OF THE HEAD, YOU WILL HEAR THE REVERBERATION OF A MOUNTAIN WATERFALL."

6:38

"THE INDWELLING SPIRIT WILL TAKE PLEASURE IN THIS VIBRATION AND IT WILL REVEAL ITSELF TO YOU."

6:39

THE KRIYA YOGA UPANISHAD, TRANSLATION BY GOSWAMI KRIYANANDA.

Sacred Waters

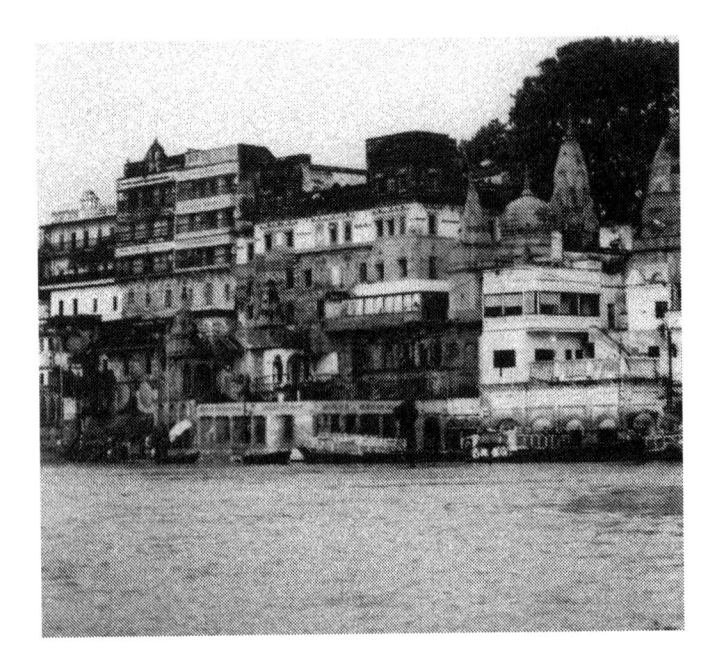

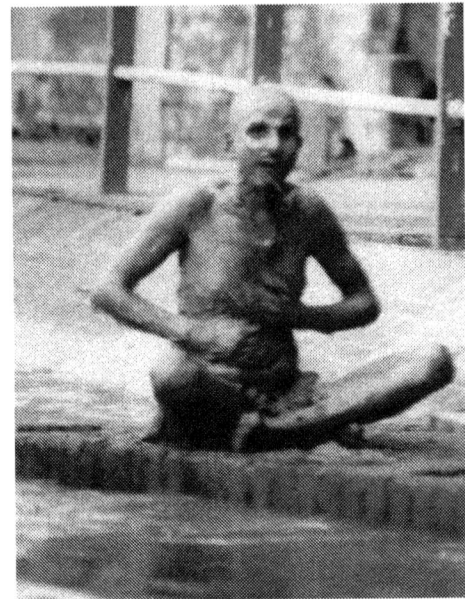

The Earth life and the Spiritual life are one and the same. The average person can become very disinterested about the source of food and water, but those civilizations that live more humbly than we do in the West, recognize and revere water as being sacred. Life typically goes on in, and around it. Water from the sacred rivers like the Ganges in particular, are collected and taken to homes and Temples the world over to be used in special blessings. The Gayatri mantra is one of the most sacred of mantras, and traditionally is chanted standing in the water at sunrise. It recognizes the indwelling Reality that is within us all.

Om Bhur bhuvaha Swaha
Tat Savitur Varenyam.
Bhargo Devasya Dhimahi
Dhiyo Yo Naha Prachodayat.
(Let's meditate on the glory of That effulgent Reality in whom the whole
universe is projected. May it enlighten our minds.)

In October, Diwali is celebrated with many tiny lamp offerings in makeshift leaf boats floating along the Ganges. The next day is a food festival honoring Annapurna. (a consort of Shiva) It is believed that evoking her presence, the entire world will be fed as she is the feeder of the world. Veranassi is the pilgrimage destination of the Hindu's who would aim to visit the Ganges at least once in a lifetime.

We are all equal in the eyes of God. Lahiri Mahasaya, a guru in the Kriya Lineage, in Yogananda's, "Autobiography of a yogi", is said to have witnessed Babaji (Lahiri's Guru and fountain head of the Lineage) washing the feet of a renunciate. It is the symbol of humility, as is touching the feet of one's guru or teacher. The symbolism is one of attunement to the astral body that is considered to be upside down to the physical body. Thus, touching the feet you are really touching his head and attuning to that level of consciousness.

Carl Jung, in "Dreams", suggests that the sea is a symbol of the collective unconscious because waters run deeper than we can know just by looking at it's surface. Once we start to walk the spiritual path consciously, many intuitive insights often come to mind. During a speech where he was explaining Christ consciousness or self-realization, apparently Lahiri cried out, "I am drowning in the bodies of many souls off the coast of Japan". It came to pass as his disciples read the next day, and is an example of our interconnectedness to all life.

In the bathing ghats along sacred Indian rivers, one can see bodies being openly cremated and their ashes then being offered to the water. To the yogi there is only death of the physical body. The soul lives on, just in another form.

"The morning sun pierced the waters; I purified myself in the Ganges, as though for a sacred initiation"
Yogananda's original Autobiography

Stepping into the Ganges means one is embracing the Divine cycle of life and death whenever it comes. Even in death there is a sense of expansion into another realm of consciousness beyond what the ordinary mind conceives of. I remember in the movie 'A passage to India', the gist of Mrs Moore's comment when she saw a dead body floating by, "Oh ! how dreadful.....how wonderful".

SACRED WATERS

"WHILE THE ROSE BLOWS ALONG THE RIVER BRINK
WITH OLD KHAYYAM THE RUBY VINTAGE DRINK;
AND WHEN THE ANGEL WITH HIS DARKER DRAUGHT
DRAWS UP TO THEE - TAKE THAT, AND DO NOT SHRINK".

OMAR KHAYYAM

The Rose is said to be Divine Bliss and the River is the pranic energies contained within the subtle spine. Old Khayyam is the transmission of wisdom and consciousness by the guru or spiritual teacher. The ruby vintage refers to the wine of ecstasy with the celestial messenger of cosmic consciousness being the Angel. Darker draught is the inner truth that comes from experience of life, and is without doubts or fears. Trust your intuition as you expand in cosmic consciousness. Do not shrink but have courage and strength.

(taken and adapted from Yogananda's explanation of Rubaiyat, which was edited by Donald Walters)

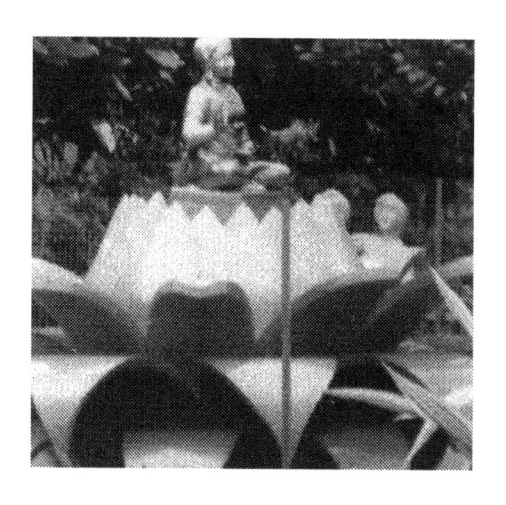

OM MANE PADME HUM

THE JEWEL IS IN THE LOTUS OF THE HEART.

THOU AND I ARE ONE

"THY COSMIC LIFE AND I ARE ONE
THOU ART THE OCEAN AND
I AM THE WAVE;
WE ARE ONE"

WHISPERS FROM ETERNITY - PARAMAHANSA YOGANANDA

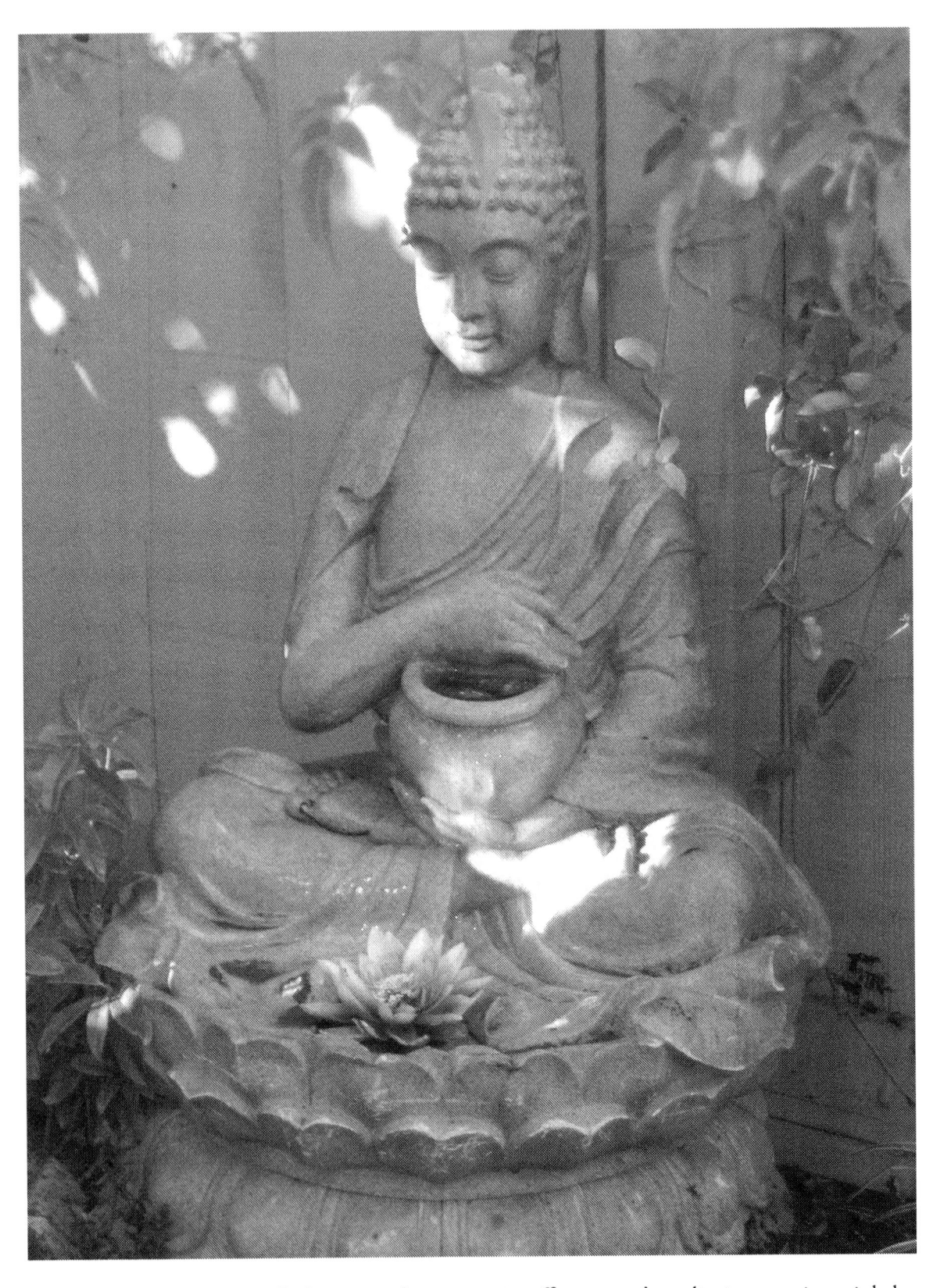

The sight, sound, or smell of water can have a positive effect on one's meditation practice as it helps us to become more aware of the subtle body and stabilize the mindstuff.

Aqua Yoga and Meditation

"Ah!" to be by the ocean and listen to its incessant roar crashing on the beaches. The waves may be pounding the beach on a gross level, but more subtly in the mind, the very thoughts we think can be beaten to submission and stillness. Beyond the desire to think any particular thought. The moods of the ocean, like nature and the human mind, are fickle and changeable, and dependant upon time, place and circumstance. Choosing a place to meditate by the water needs careful consideration. Noisy, crowded beaches during peak season are obviously not the best times to sit and meditate, but sunrise and sunset can be magical. It is best not to use words to describe the experience because that would limit it, but it is during special quiet times in nature that we can deepen our inner practice. I remember being at a yoga retreat outside Chicago. It had a lovely lake in the grounds. At the start of the retreat, the activity of the lake was turbulent, like that of the chattering students, but by the end of the weekend, the lake was like a pool of glass reflecting the re-wired minds of the group. A Kabbalistic meditation technique involves gazing at water, for in it's reflection is said to be the highest, deepest dimension of the Self.

A while ago, I was practicing some meditating overlooking the ocean in Mexico, and just as I opened my eyes, a whale appeared in my view and closed the space between it, and the meditation I had just left. A very uplifting experience, and one that looking at a picture of a whale or the ocean could not have evoked within my soul. The proximity to the salty ocean, and its spray help to clear nasal passages, and sinuses. Just licking the lips and tasting the salty water can help to stimulate the gastric juices necessary for digestion. Being by the ocean is a real feast for the senses. Salty tears running down the face, release inner tension and sadness that sometimes is a necessary part of managing our emotions, perhaps releasing grief. Time by the sea can be very healing on many levels.

"After a two hour flood of tears, I felt singularly transformed, as if by
some alchemical cleanser". - Yogananda's original Autobiography

Tratak, the act of bringing tears to the eyes, stimulates the energy centers in the brain, bringing the mind to focus on one single point. It involves adopting a nice smooth, controlled, breathing patterning, centering on a chosen object until tears flow. Then closing the eyes, still visualizing the object, one concentrates on that at the pineal gland between the eyebrows. This is known as the third eye or eye of Shiva. This is the only gland in the body that responds to light, and converts that energy to help govern the bodies glandular system. It is known as the point of transformation for the yogi.

There are many techniques that can be used in moving towards a meditative state by the water, but first a steady seated posture needs to be found. Next, try to sit with a straight spine and close your eyes. Don't try to breathe, just let the breath breathe you, and be the observer of it.

Listen to the sound of the water, and let it fill the space in the head until there is nothing but that sound. Let all other thoughts be gently pushed aside as they come into the mind. Sit for as long as you feel comfortable, and when you open your eyes, just sit for a while longer, saying and doing nothing.

The conch shell is used as an instrument delivering the sacred sound of emanation, and can send shivers down the spine before meditation. They are a true gift from the sea.

The symbolism of water and how is flows through life can be a metaphor for how we need to adapt to life, and the many challenges we are faced with. Our ancestors were very often prescribed by doctors to go and spend time at the seaside or at a spa. Alas, lots of beaches are awash with people imposing their form of recreation and noise pollution on everyone else, but secret, special places can still be found, far from the madding crowds.

Meditation at the beach

Find a quiet spot where you will be undisturbed. Adopt a comfortable seated posture with a straight spine and take a while to become still and quiet, relax the face muscles, the jaw and the tongue and listen to the sound of the sea. The lapping waves swaying back and forth in a gentle rolling motion. Inhale as the tide moves out dissolving this moment, and exhale as the waves roll in, projecting it's energy forwards from the vast abyss of the ocean, as far as the inner eye can see. Imagine the abundance of life forms under the blanket of the waves. A chalice of wonder, vibrating and alive and yet barely understood by earth man. Dive deep into this ocean and dare to dream the dream.

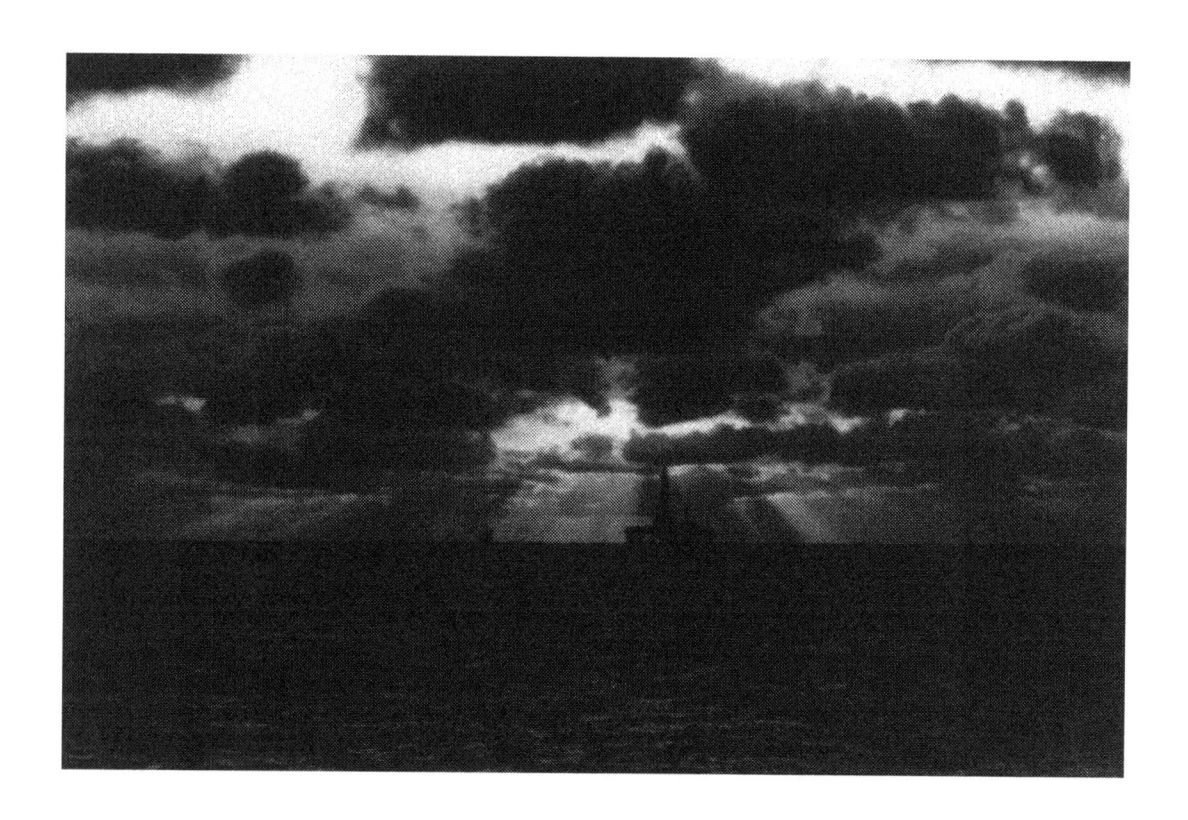

Meditation or reflection out to sea in the North, North sea in November.

Yogananda often used his observations of the ocean to teach the way to know God to many of his disciples and devotees. We tend to think of ourselves as separate from one another, like the waves in the ocean and forget that we are a part of the ocean itself. To know a drop of water is to know the whole ocean. If we can come to know ourselves, we know the anguish and joy of all mankind.

The earth life and the spiritual life are one and the same.

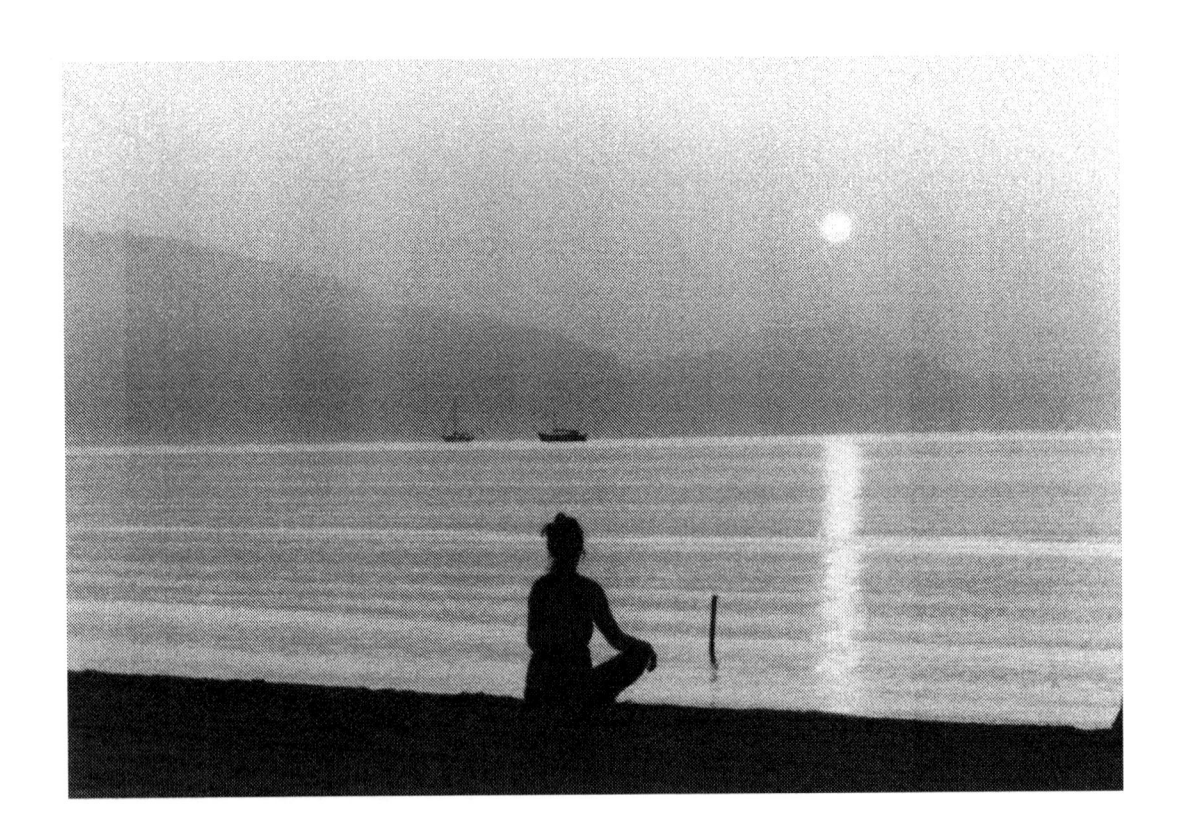

"THE YOGI MOUNTS THE CHARIOT-CAR OF AUMM, HIS CHARIOTEER IS THE LORD OF SUSTAINMENT, AND HE SEEKS THE ABODE OF THE REALITY-WORLD TO WIN FOR HIMSELF THE PRODUCTION OF SPIRITUAL RAIN: LORD SHIVA'S POWER TO DISSOLVE THE NEGATIVE KARMA THROUGH THAT HOLY CLEANSING RAIN".

THE AMRITA BINDU UPANISHAD (AMRITA NADA)

TRANSLATION BY GOSWAMI KRIYANANDA

The Maha (great) asana is learning to stand on your own two feet.........Goswami Kriyananda

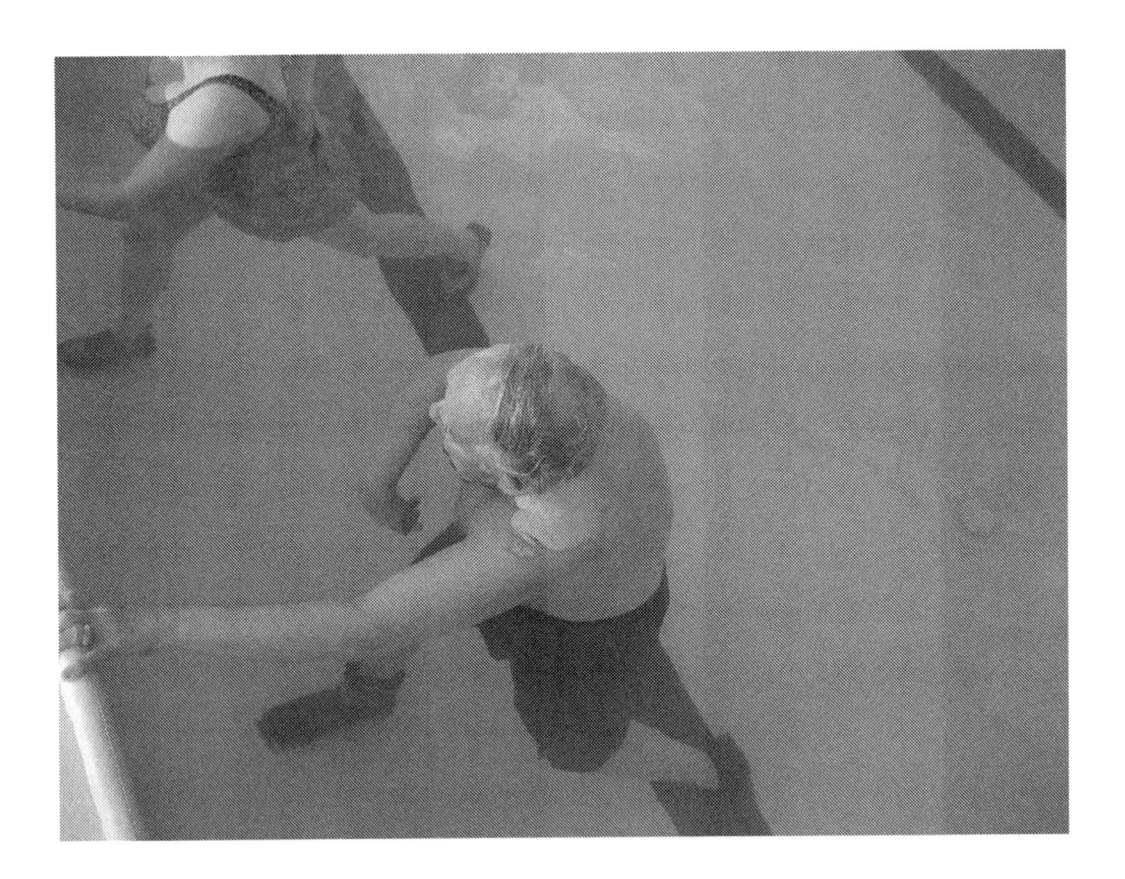

It may be possible and psychologically beneficial for some people with balance issues or who are normally confined to a wheel chair to physically try and stand on their on two feet. (Please understand that this is an internal destination rather than a destination in place and time.)

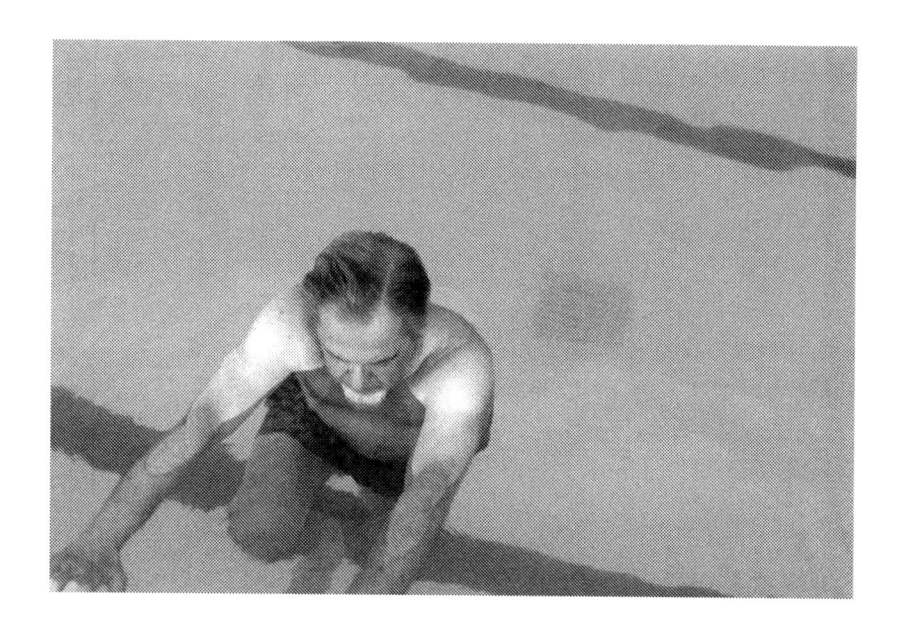

Acknowledgements:

For spiritual teaching:
Goswami Kriyananda - Temple of Kriya Yoga – Chicago
Swami Enoch Dasa Giri - Temple of Kriya Yoga – Chicago

For opportunity to teach Aqua Yoga – Saratoga YMCA   C.A.

For their blessings and inspiration - My students.
For believing in the book and encouraging me to get it published - Dasaji and Kenny.

For the creative environment living, at Ananda.

For Julie's selfless service on the computer.

Contact information;

camyoga@gmail.com
www.camellayoga.org
www.yogakriya.org
www.liliasyoga.com
www.ipdtransform.com

Suggested Further Reading

"Spiritual Science of Kriya Yoga", obtained from the Temple.

"Yoga Gets Better With Age", Lilias Folan

Available from Camella's website -

www.camellayoga.org or e-mail to camyoga@gmail.com

CD AUM chant, "Om Hatha Sadhana", 85 mins
Pricing: $15.00 (plus shipping and handling)

Gayatri and other mantras available from camella's website or e-mail directly.

Kriology home study program – Obtained from the Temple www.yogakriya.org

Workshops and retreats

For beginners or intermediates on land/water contact Camella camyoga@gmail.com

Bibliography:

"Water Dance" by Juliana Larson
"The Yoga of Nutrition" Omram Nikhael Aivanton
"Dhanwantari" Harish Johari
"Varanasi" DR. Raj Bali Pandey
"Meditations and Mantras" Swami Vishnu Devananda
"King Arthur Dark Age Warrior and Mythic Hero" John Mattews
"Vastu Shastra" Caroline Robertson
" The Essential Kabbalah " Daniel C.Matt
"Autobiography of a Yogi" Yogananda's Original Version
"God's Jewels- Their Dignity and Destiny" W.Y. Fullerton

Monsoon In India and my darling boys.

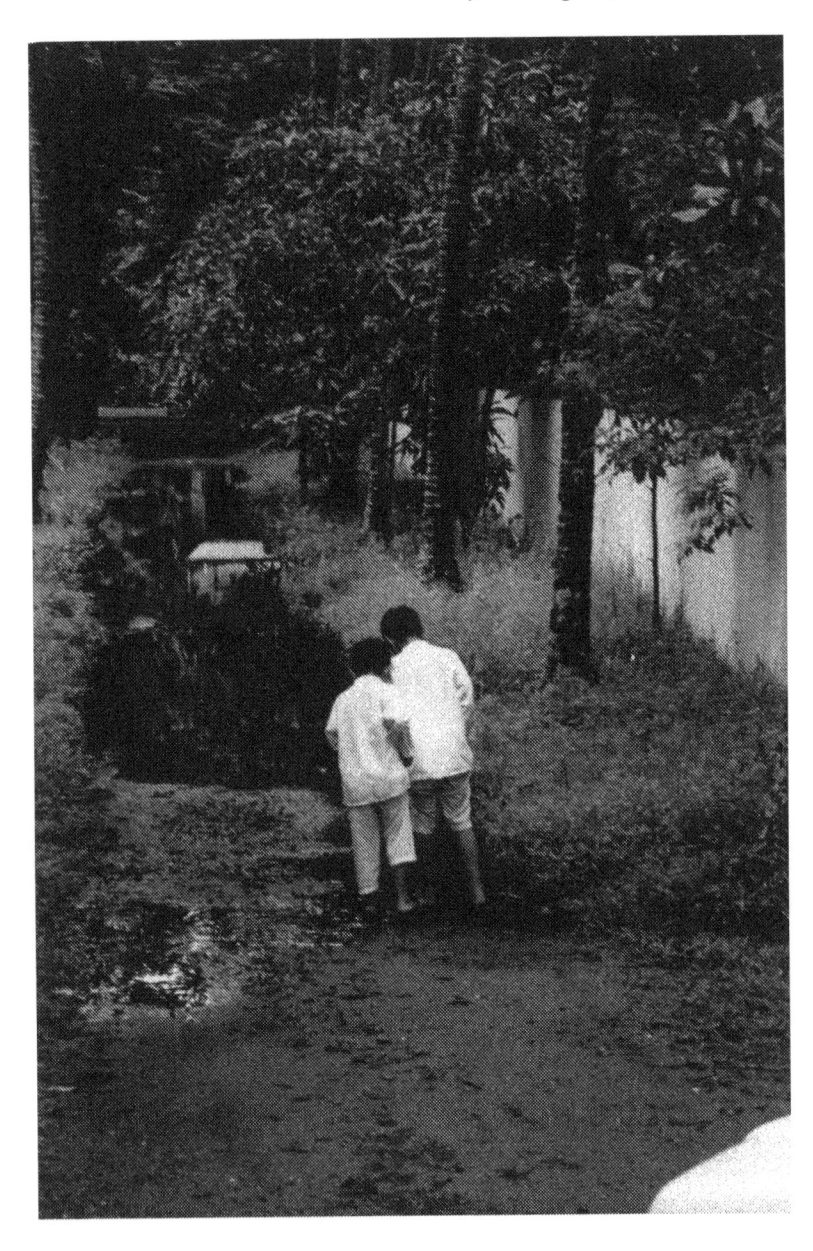

Frantic Rain

Whispering caresses as the morning breeze sweeps across my well slumbered cheek as I assume the asana of contemplation.

The gentle ripple of vrittis merge, and get swallowed up whole into the mouth of Mother Nature, as tho' water pours through a strainer into the canopy above.

What vastness of reserves the sky doth harbor in its bosom, all to be violently released at the flick of a switch.

Five minutes hence, the crashing crescendo abaits as suddenly as it began. Then...brief silence.

An all too brief reprieve as the 'putt-putt' engines start in the distance. Ready ! set! go ! Krishna's song now fully restored in God's misty steam room.

Then deluge. Pounding, frantic rain, trying to outdo the previous shower.

Drenching everything it touches as it beats to the rhythm of the Monsoon,
prizing open the lids of privacy after a rush of energy swirls around Chandra. The fervent fever demanding center stage as she cloaks the swaying palms with a gossamer shroud.

Then silence once more.

A sharp intake of breath as the spoiled waters from beneath the Earth's crust
pierce the senses.

The scudding clouds are wisped away like a child's hastily drawn "etch a
Sketch", revealing strands of baby blue.

A jackdaw crows, calling out to fellow revelers to take flight now. Their instinctive knowingness taking heed of the dark clouds to the east, reading their dance like the pages of a well loved book.

A lone black fly takes it's chances and goads me into action as it settles on this vessels glossy thigh.

The meditation is over once more. Or maybe now it's just begun.

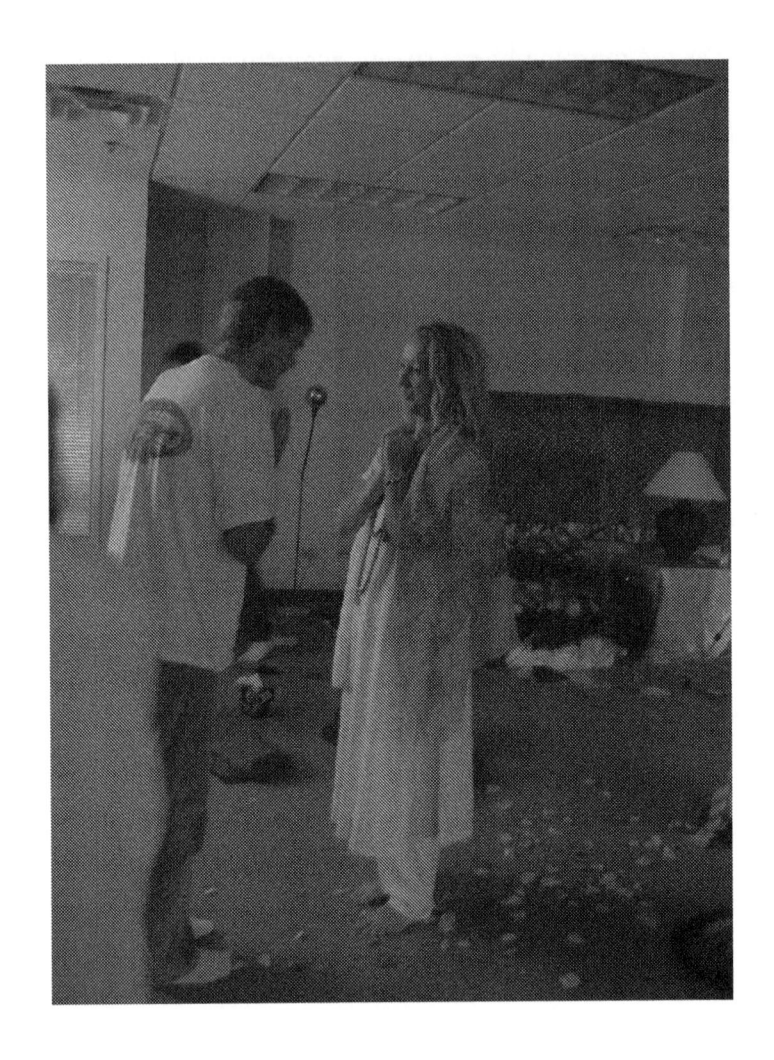

Camella Nair R.Y.T (Swami Nibhrtananda)

Camella has been practicing yoga for over 25 years and has made yoga accessible to those who may never step into a yoga class on land, whilst giving the experienced yogi another medium in which to explore the ancient science of yoga.

She currently teaches many styles of yoga covering a wide range of students in the South Bay area of Northern California. She can be contacted by e-mail.

Lightning Source UK Ltd.
Milton Keynes UK
UKHW050904131021
392109UK00002B/17

9 781434 334046